CHINESE QIGONG ACUPRESSURE THERAPY

A Traditional Healing Technology for the Modern World

Huang Xiaokuan

FOREIGN LANGUAGES PRESS   BEIJING

First Edition 1997

Translated by Wang Tai

ISBN 7-119-00748-3

© Foreign Languages Press, Beijing, 1997
Published by Foreign Languages Press
24 Baiwanzhuang Road, Beijing 100037, China

Printed by Foreign Languages Printing House
19 Chegongzhuang Xilu, Beijing 100044, China

Distributed by China International Book Trading Corporation
35 Chegongzhuang Xilu, Beijing 100044, China
P.O. BOX 399, Beijing, China

Printed in the People's Republic of China

CONTENTS

Foreword   1

Chapter 1
Qigong Acupressure Therapy Basics   3
  What Is Qigong Acupressure Therapy   3
  Scope and Effects of Qigong Acupressure Therapy   3
  Characteristics of Qigong Acupressure Therapy   4
  Therapeutic Mechanism of Qigong Acupressure Therapy   4
  Healing Applications and Contraindications of Qigong Acupressure Therapy   5
  Times and Courses of Qigong Acupressure Therapy   6
  How to Learn and Practise Qigong Acupressure Therapy   7
  Cautions and Comments   7

Chapter 2
Qigong Acupressure Therapy Exercises   9
  Preliminary Exercise   9
  Shaolin Post-Standing   9
  Robust Man Squatting and Standing-Up   11
  Patting the Dantian   11
  Strengthening the Loins and Tonifying the Kidneys   12
  Slapping with Cinnabar Palm   13
  Taiji Ball   14
  Erlang Immortal Carrying Mount Taishan   15
  Pushing-Up with Dragon's Claws   15
  Palm-Pushing with Potential Strength   17
  Boy Worshiping the Buddha   18
  Closing Posture   18

Chapter 3
Supplemental Qigong Acupressure Therapy Exercises   20
  Weight Control and Calisthenics   20
  Eight Pieces of Brocade Exercise   24
  Eye Healing Techniques   29

Chapter 4
Basic Qigong Acupressure Therapy Techniques   33
   Pressing   33
   Vibrating   34
   Knocking   35
   Patting   35
   Grasping   37
   Kneading   38
   Push-Rubbing   40
   Rolling   42

Chapter 5
Location and Healing Applications of Common Acupoints and Clinical Formulae   44
   Concept of Meridians and Acupoints   44
   Courses and Acupoints of the 14 Meridians   45
   Common Acupoints for Qigong Acupressure   47
   Acupoint Formulae for Qigong Acupressure Therapy   60

Chapter 6
Clinical Practice of Qigong Acupressure Therapy   65
   Essentials of Qigong Acupressure Therapy   65
   Therapeutic Methods for Different Syndromes   66
   Qigong Acupressure Therapy on Different Parts of the Body   66
      Qigong Acupressure Therapy on the Head   66
      Qigong Acupressure Therapy on the Neck   67
      Qigong Acupressure Therapy on the Chest and Abdomen   68
      Qigong Acupressure Therapy on the Back and Lumbar Regions   69
      Qigong Acupressure Therapy on the Four Limb Joints   70
   Qigong Acupressure Therapy for Common Diseases   70
      Headaches   71
      Vertigo   72
      Fainting   73
      Asthma   75
      Insomnia   76
      Vomiting   77
      Hiccups   78
      Toothaches   79
      Myopia   80

Stiff Necks   81
Periarthritis of the Shoulder   82
Cervical Spondylopathy   83
Chest and Rib Pain   85
Stomachaches   86
Abdominal Pain   88
Constipation   90
Heat Stroke   91
Dysmenorrhea   92
Paralysis   93
Emission   95
Impotence   96
Mastitis   97
Intestinal Obstructions   97
Diabetes Mellitus   98
Lumbago   100
Rheumatoid Arthritis   101
Calf Muscle Spasms   103
Rheumatic Arthritis of the Knee Joint   104
Ankle Injuries   105
Arm Sprains and Contusions   106
Lower Limb Sprains and Contusions   107
Postencephalitis   108
Cerebral Palsy   110
Hemiplegia   111
Traumatic Paraplegia   113
Bed-Wetting (Enuresis)   115
Infantile Indigestion   116
Myogenic Torticollis in Children   117

FOREWORD

Qigong acupressure therapy is an important branch of traditional Chinese medicine which specializes in using breathing and movement exercises to cultivate health and treat diseases. It contains the accumulated knowledge and clinical experience of many dynasties. The therapeutic techniques of qigong acupressure therapy are simple and easy to learn and practise and do not rely on drugs or medical equipment and does not produce side effects. Qigong acupressure therapy can be used to treat many common diseases: hypertension, coronary heart disease, peptic ulcer, diabetes mellitus, neurasthenia, pulmonary fibrosis and neck, shoulder, lower back and leg pains. It also has produced some exciting results with difficult and complicated diseases such as hemiplegia, paraplegia and cancers.

The author of the book began to learn and regularly perform Shaolin internal qigong from his young age; and stemmed from his good spirit to study and work hard and adeptly, he already obtained rich knowledge and experience from clinical practice of qigong acupressure therapy. This book sums up his many years of clinical experience and scientific research, and is an excellent reference manual for healing professionals and amateurs.

Guo Wuyi

Vice-president of College for
Advanced Chinese Qigong

October 3, 1994

Chapter 1
QIGONG ACUPRESSURE THERAPY BASICS

What Is Qigong Acupressure Therapy

Qigong acupressure therapy is a particular form of qigong therapy. According to the nature and severity of diseases, common techniques of massage, such as finger-pressing, vibrating, knocking, patting, grasping, kneading, push-rubbing and rolling are used to stimulate appropriate acupoints, meridians or special places on the body surface. Therapists use their hands (or other body parts), reinforced by concentrated qi, to promote circulation of qi and blood in the body and to restore normal functioning of impaired organs. This mode of treatment is called qigong acupressure therapy because fingers or palms are used to apply pressure with concentrated qi to acupoints or meridians for curing diseases.

Qi is always applied in combination with concentration and awareness to the acupoint. Qigong acupressure with concentrated qi to cure diseases is a complicated therapeutic technique: it can only be practised by a few qualified qigong experts.

Scope and Effects of Qigong Acupressure Therapy

Qigong acupressure is a medical application of the qigong and martial arts (*gongfu*) practised in ancient China. Qigong acupressure therapy contains the same finger-pressing, hitting, grasping and kicking techniques used by martial artists to attack enemies and protect themselves from injury. Qigong acupressure skillfully transfers this knowledge to the medical field to treat diseases.

Nowadays, qigong acupressure is widely used in Chinese medical clinics and is welcomed by the masses because of its simple techniques, good results and lack of side-effects. Through many years of clinical practice (treating over 10,000 patients), rich knowledge and experience have accumulated about its healing applications.

We have had excellent clinical results with patients suffering from paralysis, cervical spondylosis, periarthritis of the shoulder, prolapse of lumbar vertebral disc, arthropathy of limbs, gastrointestinal neurosis, insomnia, neurasthenia, diabetes mellitus, hypertrophy of prostate gland, andropathy and cancers. For example, the cure rate was 89 percent in 68 cases of hemiplagia and paraplegia; 100 percent total effectiveness rate and 78 percent excellence rate in 61 cases of junior myopia; 89 percent total effectiveness rate and 78 percent excellence rate in 60 cases of neurasthenia; 100 percent total effectiveness rate and 95 percent excellence rate in 40 cases of pain syndrome; 100 percent total effectiveness rate and 88 percent excellence rate in 72 cases of gynecological diseases; 90 percent total effectiveness rate and 61 percent excellence rate in 106 cases of lower back and leg pain; 96 percent total effectiveness rate and 81 percent excellence rate in 218 cases of soft tissue injury; and 96 percent total effectiveness rate and 77 percent excellence rate in 48 cases of soft tissue injury of neck and arm.

Characteristics of Qigong Acupressure Therapy

Qigong acupressure is a therapeutic to cure diseases by applying thermal energy, derived from concentrated qi to the meridians, joints, nerves and blood vessels on the body surface by means of various techniques of massage. It may adjust neural and humoral functions and balance yin and yang in the body to cure disease. The characteristics of qigong acupressure are as follows:

1. Wide applications: Qigong acupressure is useful to treat many diseases, belonging to different branches of medicine, but it is most effective in treating patients with chronic functional disturbance or those in the recovery stage. For example, it may produce a good results in chronic patients with paralysis.

2. Simple to learn and practise: In general, beginners may use it for clinical practice after studying hard for three to five months.

3. Safety and effectiveness: It is a safe, comfortable and effective treatment for many internal and external diseases, but the application of pressure and qi to the acupoints should be adequate in intensity.

4. Easy application and inexpensive: An inexpensive, simple and effective therapeutic treatment, qigong acupressure may be used anywhere and at any time. No special equipment or medical instruments are required.

5. Disease prevention and health maintenance: Once the technique of qigong acupressure therapy has been mastered, people may use it for themselves or on others to prevent diseases and maintain health.

Therapeutic Mechanism of Qigong Acupressure Therapy

Because qigong acupressure originated from ancient martial arts and traditional Chinese medicine, it should be practised following traditional Chinese medical theories and principles of diagnosis and treatment on overall analysis of the illness and the patient's condition. This therapy has been combined with modern medicine in clinical practice and its therapeutic mechanism can be explained by modern medical theories.

1. As mentioned in ancient classical medical books, the *Yellow Emperor's Canon of Medicine*: "The qi, blood, essence and spirit in human body may circulate through meridians and spread all over the body to adjust yin and yang, nourish muscles, bones and joints and save the organism's life"; and "the 12 meridians in the body can adjust the functions of five Zang Organs (five internal organs: heart, liver, spleen, lungs

and kidneys) and six Fu Organs (vital organs of the human body) to keep a harmonious coordination between the human body and surrounding environment." Under normal physiological conditions, the meridians are a network of channels for qi and blood to circulate and spread all over the body and to hold the organism as an integrated living entity; but under pathological conditions, they may transmit pathogenic factors and pathological influence between organs and structures in the body to cause imbalance between yin and yang; disturbance and stagnation of *ying* (nutrients), *wei* (defensive energy), qi and blood and finally to cause sickness. As mentioned in ancient medical books: "If the closed 'door' or 'window' of meridians can be reopened and qi and blood may recover normal circulation, then the disease can be cured. Therefore, stagnated qi, proximal to the closed segment of meridian should be led forward to overcome the obstacle by applying adequate stimulation to the appropriate acupoints." After the acupoints are stimulated by finger-pressing, vibrating, knocking, patting, grasping, kneading, push-rubbing and rolling maneuvers, the meridianal qi can be activated, the blockage of meridian can be relieved, the circulation of qi and blood can be promoted, the balance between *ying, wei*, qi and blood can be restored and the functions of internal organs can be adjusted and integrated.

2. Under normal conditions, yin and yang in the body are balanced and the functions of organs are harmonious. If the balance between yin and yang is disturbed by noxious factors the body is likely to attract illness. For example, influenza fever in children is usually caused by a deficiency in vital energy, impairment of *wei* qi (body resistance) and invasion by external wind and heat evils (pathogenic factors). As traditional Chinese physicians say, "External evils always attack people deficient in qi." The techniques of qigong acupressure deal with this situation by enhancing vital energy and expelling external evils from the body, thus maintaining health and curing diseases.

3. According to modern medicine, qigong acupressure cures diseases because it adjusts the functioning of the central nervous system, improves blood circulation and metabolism in the focus of disease and enhances the recovery and regeneration of damaged tissues of the lesion.

In brief, qigong acupressure therapy may produce multiple effects: relieving meridian blockages, promoting circulation of qi and blood, adjusting yin and yang imbalance, restoring vital energy, expelling external evils, postponing the aging process and prolonging life span.

Healing Applications and Contraindications of Qigong Acupressure Therapy

Healing Applications

Common Diseases:
Surgical Diseases: diseases of shoulder, elbow, wrist, and phalangeal joints,

cervical spondylosis, stiff neck, diseases of lower back, muscular sprain of lower back, prolapse of lumbar vertebral disc, sciatica neuralgia, soft tissue injury of buttocks, and injury of iliosacral joint.

Internal Diseases: headaches, stomachaches, neurasthenia, neurogenic vomiting, hiccups, hydrocephalus, hysteria, infantile indigestion, incontinence of urine in children, impotence, nocturnal emission, myopia, dysmenorrhea, acute gastroenteritis, heat stroke and syncope.

Complicated Diseases: cerebral hemiplegia, paraplegia, sequelae of encephalitis, polyneuritis, Bell's palsy, cerebral contusion and injury of sciatic nerve.

Other Diseases: brain tumors, cancer of the intestine, pulmonary fibrosis and qigong psychoneurosis.

Contraindications:

Acute Diseases: acute stages of inflammation, acute abdomen, febrile and infectious diseases

Serious Diseases: severe hypertension, heart disease and late stages of cancer

Hemorrhagic Diseases: hemophilia, allergic purpura and thrombocytopenic purpura

Skin Diseases: severe skin diseases

Times and Courses of Qigong Acupressure Therapy

In general, qigong acupressure may be applied once a day. A routine therapeutic course includes 6-18 treatments. In patients with mild diseases and short clinical course, a therapeutic course may contain 6-24 treatments. In chronic patients, a therapeutic course may last for 1-3 months, and in paraplegic patients, 3-6 months. The acupressure treatment may be discontinued, if the patient's health improves enough. In order to increase the therapeutic effect, it is best if patients complete the entire therapeutic course.

The chronometric (time-related) phenomenon described in traditional medicine is quite similar to the biological clock in modern medicine and it is usually used to explain the time-related circulation of qi through the meridian system. Because the qigong acupressure therapy is applied at the acupoints of the meridians, it is of course closely related to the flow of qi through the meridian and the qigong acupressure practioners may choose an adequate time to treat the patient. For example, at noon (11-13 o'clock), i.e. Wu o'clock in Chinese chronometry qi is flowing through the Heart Meridian, it is the best time to treat patients with heart diseases by qigong acupressure therapy. The time table of qi circulation in the meridian system is shown as follows:

Chinese Clock	Western Clock	Meridian
Zi	23-1	Gallbladder
Chou	1-3	Liver

Yin	3-5	Lung
Mao	5-7	Large Intestine
Chen	7-9	Stomach
Si	9-11	Spleen
Wu	11-13	Heart
Wei	13-15	Small Intestine
Shen	15-17	Urinary Bladder
You	17-19	Kidney
Xu	19-21	Pericardium
Hai	21-23	Sanjiao

How to Learn and Practise Qigong Acupressure Therapy

1. In order to master qigong acupressure therapy, the acupoints must be kept firmly in mind and the techniques and other fundamental skills should be correctly executed and gradually improved over years of practice.

2. Qigong acupressure therapy practioners can excel if they have a forceful and robust physique and accomplished skill. There are three basic exercises to practice for fulfiling above requirement: (1) arm exercises for strengthening arm force; (2) wrist exercises for improving skillfulness and elasticity.... (3) fingers exercises for increasing firmness and endurance. A good therapeutic result can be obtained only after the concentration of thought and application of qi and pressure by the finger can be carried out simultaneously and coordinately. If the beginners want to use qigong acupressure therapy in clinic after a short training course, they are better to: (1) read hard the basic knowledge about the fundamental exercise of qigong and the therapeutic techniques of qigong acupressure in textbooks and carry on earnestly and persistently the physical exercise following the directions about the action, posture and other requirements of physical exercise emphasized in the textbooks until they are qualified; (2) carefully, seriously and preoccupiedly accomplish the performance of qigong acupressure with their visual line and finger pressure concentrated at the acupoints; and (3) select correct acupoints and adequate techniques to treat patients and watch their response to your treatment over time. A good therapeutic results can be obtained only after a successful treatment at correct acupoints with appropriate techniques to apply necessary amount of qi.

Cautions and Comments

1. Before the qigong acupressure treatment, a correct differential diagnosis of both modern and traditional medicine must be made after conscientiously collecting the information of disease and defining the exact location of lesion by careful palpation and comparison with the normal side for establishing a proper therapeutic principle and arranging a useful therapeutic program. A satisfactory therapeutic result can be obtained only after correct selection of acupoints and adequate application of therapeutic maneuvers.

2. Before the application of qigong acupressure therapy, the finger nails of physicians should be cut short to avoid any injury to the patients' skin. The pressure applied by the finger and the amount of qi delivered to the acupoints should be determined and gradually increased according to the duration of disease and the condition of patients. For example, acupressure manipulation must be very gentle in patients with chronic diseases, in starvation or after a heavy meal; qigong acupressure is prohibited in pregnant women and should be postponed in drunken or over-fatigued patients; and acupressure must be very gentle to avoid bone fracture, in patients with bone deformity.

3. After qigong acupressure therapy, most patients experience a relief of symptoms, a comfortable and relaxed feeling, sound sleep, improved appetite and increased body weight. However, some patients may show signs of a worsening condition. In general, it is only a temporary response to the treatment and may disappear after the treatment is continued for 2-3 more days. An explanation is necessary to relieve the patients' worry about the temporary setback.

4. After qigong acupressure therapy treatments, patients may feel hot, sore, numb and distending sensations around the acupoints with some local redness, heat, sweating and twitches. These are normal response to the treatment and need not cause concern: they will soon spontaneously disappear. In some patients acupressure may produce ecchymoses, which will also spontaneously subside after one week. If patients develop severe side effects, such as dizziness, nausea, pale complexion or syncope, nail-pinching at the nasal septum or base of finger nails or toes may help relieve these reactions.

5. Treatment of complications: (1) Temporary arrest of respiration caused by extraordinary strong stimulation of acupressure applied over the back may be relieved by patting with concentrated qi over the neck, shoulder and back, by finger-pressing with concentrated qi at Yaoyan (EX-B 7) or by grasping abdominal oblique muscles. (2) Temporary weakness or paralysis of the arm caused by extraordinary strong stimulation applied over the scapular region may be relieved by patting with concentrated qi over the shoulder, elbow or wrist. (3) Temporary weakness or paralysis of the leg caused by extraordinary strong stimulation over the lateral side of buttocks may be relieved by patting with concentrated qi over the lower back, buttocks and popliteal fossa.

Chapter 2
QIGONG ACUPRESSURE THERAPY EXERCISES

The basic exercises for qigong acupressure therapy contain ten exercises (sections), derived from Chinese qigong. They include external (physical) and internal (mental) *dangong* (exercise of qi from Dantian). It is a combination of traditional dynamic and static exercise that developed based on traditional Chinese medical theory and clinical practice. These exercises are very useful for qigong practioners and also helpful to qigong amateurs to improve their health and prevent disease. The exercises are simple, easy to learn, and produce quick results. For maintaining health and curing chronic diseases the performers may either do a complete exercise set or select a few postures suitable to their physique or useful for treating their condition.

Preliminary Exercise

The therapeutic effect of qigong acupressure is chiefly determined by the practioner's degree of internal power (internal qi or potential energy). Although it is invisible, the qi's electric shock-like sensation can be detected by patients as it deeply penetrates into the bones and internal organs. The patient may feel a hot and numb sensation spread all over their body. Before performing this set of ten exercises, perform this preliminary exercise to generate vital qi: watch straight forward, keep your mind quiet, slightly close your mouth, gently touch your upper palate with the tip of your tongue, let your elbows hang down, relax your shoulders and stretch your back. Breath smoothly and evenly, relaxing whole body and concentrating mental attention at the Dantian (an anatomical location in lower abdomen).

Shaolin Post-Standing

Basic Instructions: This exercise teaches you to stand straight as a post. Squat down with the thighs lowered to an almost horizontal level and the limbs widely stretched out. Throughout the exercise, stand with the feet parallel, three foot-lengths apart. The knees are bent with the thighs lowered down to an almost horizontal level. The toes of the feet turn slightly inward and stuck to the ground firmly with the body's centre of gravity directly above the middle point between both feet. Then, the knees turn slightly outward with the toes pointing forward. The crotch must be round and solid and the neck is kept straight; the shoulders are dropped; the elbows are bent and held in front of the chest, and the palms are turned over to face the ground with the thumbs widely separated apart from the index fingers. The other fingers are slightly separated from each other and the middle fingers opposite to each other. The arms are raised to shoulder level, and the eyes looking forward to the middle fingers. Before finishing the exercise, put the hands on Dantian for a while and then drop the hands on both sides naturally (Fig. 2-1).

The exercise may be divided into several segments and pauses. Each segment should not be less than 3-5 minutes and the whole exercise should not take less than 30 minutes. At the second step of the exercise, the standing posture is maintained and draw the arms back to the chest and then push them forward repeatedly in coordination with the respiratory movement. Inhale when draw the arms back and exhale when push the arms forward. At the same time, the qi of Dantian is kneaded, moved upward and pressed down using the imagination. The second step of exercise may be continued for 3 minutes (Fig. 2-2).

Health Benefits: The Shaolin Post-Standing Exercise is a combination of internal (mental) and external (physical) exercise to reinforce the strength of legs for keeping a stable posture and sticking the feet to the ground (solid effect) and to improve the spring force of lower limbs. Consistent practice can help maintain a good body posture, reinforce the muscular strength of arm, lower back and hip, improve the flexibility of body and it can also strengthen the waist, tonify the kidney and enrich Dantian qi.

Healing Applications: It is very useful to treat neurasthenia, insomnia and lower back pain, legs and lower limb joints.

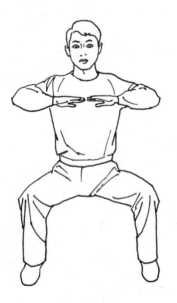
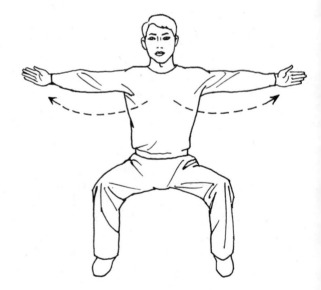

Fig. 2-1 Shaolin Post-Standing Exercise   Fig. 2-2 Shaolin Post-Standing Exercise

Robust Man Squatting and Standing-Up

Basic Instructions: Stand with feet shoulder width apart, weight evenly distributed. Then, squat down with both hands clenched and elbows bent (Figs. 2-3, 4), and then stand up. The Dantian qi is concentrated and transferred to fists and feet and the attention of mind is concentrated in the palms and then moved through the Dantian and legs to the feet. The breath should be even, smooth and keep pace with the movement of the body. The exercise may be repeated 9-18 times.

Health Benefits: This exercise can strengthen the muscles, bones and waist, tonify the kidney and reinforce the strength and endurance of the body.

Healing Applications: Arthritis, kidney diseases, emission, impotence, indigestion and emphysema of lungs.

Patting the Dantian

Basic Instructions: Patting Dantian exercise is a modification of a patting exercise of *xingyi* (figure and mind) shadow boxing, an important branch of martial arts, developed from ancient times. Assume the Shaolin Post-Standing posture, then raise the arms over the head with the palms facing down; then move the arms downward from the chest to Dantian with the palms crossed. At the same time, imagine that the yang qi collected from heaven and the yin qi received from earth are transported to middle Dantian [1.5 cun (a universal length unit used in acupuncture) below umbilicus] and the mixed qi is transferred to and condensed in the Dantian (Fig. 2-5).

This exercise may also be performed in another way: the arms are raised

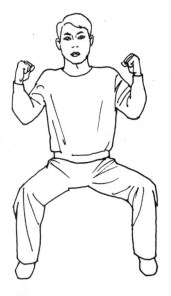

Fig. 2-3 Robust Man Squatting and
Standing-up Exercise

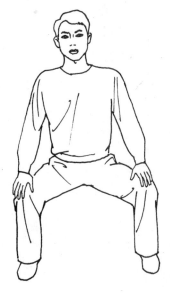

Fig. 2-4 Robust Man Squatting and
Standing-up Exercise

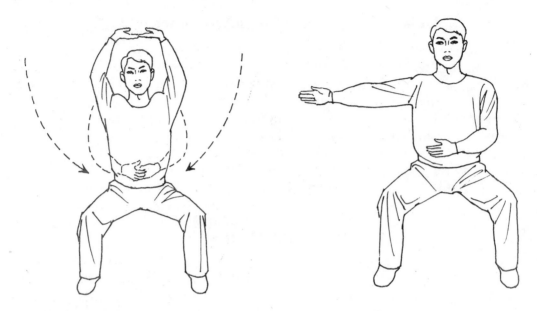

Fig. 2-5 Gathering Qi to the Dantian Exercise   Fig. 2-6 Gathering Qi to the Dantian Exercise

horizontally to the lateral side of body with palms turned up and fingers separated from each other, then the left and right palms are used to alternately pat the abdomen (Fig. 2-6), and finally, place the left hand overlapped by the right on the abdomen and rest the awareness on the Dantian for a while. Beginners may perform the exercise with natural respiration, keeping pace with the movement of exercise and experts may adopt abdominal respiration. Repeat 9-18 times.

Health Benefits: The yang qi from heaven and yin qi from earth may adjust yin and yang in the body and maintain the balance between them. This exercise can enrich Dantian qi, strengthen the spleen and stomach, reinforce the loins and tonify the kidney.

Healing Applications: Poor appetite, indigestion, incontinence of urine and stool, bed-wetting, emission, impotence and paralysis of abdominal muscles.

Strengthening the Loins and Tonifying the Kidneys

Basic Instructions: Assume the Shaolin Post-Standing Posture, the arms draw a circle as they move from the abdomen through the armpit. Qi is collected and led to the lower back region using the fingers of both hands. Then qi is introduced into the posterior Dantian (life gate) by touching and pressing the kidney region with both hands. The movement of qi is guided by concentrated mental awareness. Repeat 9-18 times. Natural respiration should be maintained (Fig. 2-7).

The same exercise may be performed in another way. After taking the Shaolin Post-Standing Posture, stand with the back straight, leaning against a wall or a tree.

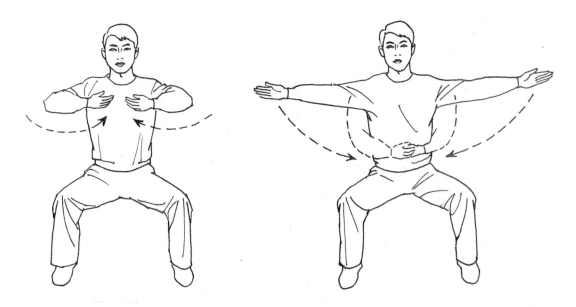

Fig. 2-7 Strengthening the Loins and Tonifying   Fig. 2-8 Strengthening the Loins with Back
          the Kidneys Exercise   Against a Wall Exercise

The chest is expanded by stretching and swinging the arms back and forth with the back hitting the wall gently, producing a shaking sensation in the spinal column and to promoting circulation of qi and blood through the Du Meridian and over the back region. Repeat 9-18 times (Fig. 2-8).

Health Benefits: The exercise can promote circulation of qi and blood through the back and Du meridian, reinforce muscular strength in the back and loins and tonify the kidney. If this exercise is consistantly practised over a long period of time, the shoulders, back and waist will become strong, muscular and firm.

Healing Applications: Back pain and lumbago, paralysis of nerves, improving health and building up powerful physique.

Slapping with Cinnabar Palm

Basic Instructions: This name refers to the redness of the palm due to the presence of qi; cinnabor (zhusha) is a red-colored herb used in Chinese medicine. Assuming the post-standing posture, raise the arms forward to shoulder height (keeping shoulder-distance) with the palms facing forward and the thumbs facing each other (Fig. 2-9). Qi is transferred from lower Dantian through upper Dantian to inner Laogong (PC 8) at the centers of the palms. The palms, with concentrated qi, are slowly pushed forward until the arms fully extended or against some obstacles. For example, first use a paper board and later replace it with a wooden board, then with a stone plate and finally with an iron plate (Fig. 2-10). The forward push of

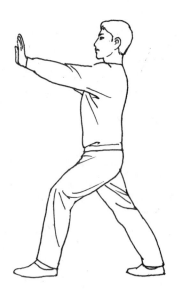 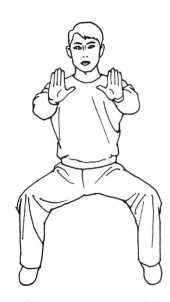

Fig. 2-9 Slapping with Zhusha Palm Exercise   Fig. 2-10 Slapping with Zhusha Palm Exercise

palms should be reinforced by exhalation and the backward withdrawal of the palms aided by inhalation of air. Mental awareness is kept concentrated on the palms and coordinated with the movement of the palms. Both palms may move forward and backward simultaneously or alternately 9-18 times.

Health Benefits: This exercise can strengthen the arms, palms and fingers and improve the range of motion in the arms.

Healing Applications: The exercise can be used to treat functional impairment of joints of arm and during this exercise, internal qi is concentrated in the fingers and then released to produce external qi which can be used for qigong acupressure therapy.

Taiji Ball

Basic Instructions: Assume the Shaolin Post-Standing Posture, and hold a round sand bag of 3.5 kg in weight in each hand. Circle the arms from left to right beside the body and then raise them up and down for more than 100 times (Fig. 2-11). Finally, rotate the ball in the palm more than 100 times (Fig. 2-12). The exercise may be repeated 9-18 times in one session.

· Health Benefits: The performance of this exercise seems not violent and energy-consumed, but it may produce a remarkable effect to enrich internal qi and reinforce the strength of the arms, palms and fingers.

Healing Applications: This is a useful exercise for functional recovery of injured arms, such as constrictive capsulitis of shoulder and cervical spondylosis. After

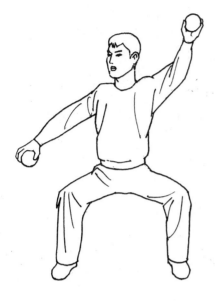 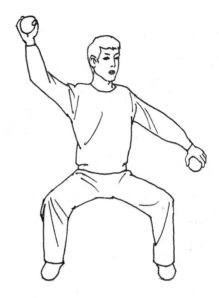

Fig. 2-11 Taiji Ball Exercise   Fig. 2-12 Taiji Ball Exercise

continuous practice over a long period of time, practioners may be able to move Dantion qi to the palms and fingers and use it to treat patients with qigong acupressure.

Erlang Immortal Carrying Mount Taishan

Basic Instructions: Assume a post-standing posture, and transfer Dantian qi to both arms and palms. Stretch the arms laterally, pushing out the palms to both sides. At the same time, concentrated awareness is guided through the medial side of arms to inner Laogong (PC 8) in the palms. Shake the arms up and down and turn the palms over, assuming a supporting gesture as if you were trying to carry Mount Taishan with a shoulder pole (Fig. 2-13). Repeat 9-18 times.

Health Benefits: The exercise can strengthen the arms and wrists, incerase Dantian qi and internal strength and improve one's physique and general health.

Healing Applications: The exercise may prevent and treat cervical spondylosis, constrictive capsulitis and pain in the lower back and legs. It may also provide rich qi for qigong acupressure therapy.

Pushing-Up with Dragon's Claws

Basic Instructions: Lie prostate on the floor with the chest, abdomen and legs above the floor, and the palms and toes touching the floor to support the body. Then, straighten back as shown in the diagrams (Figs. 2-14, 2-15 and 2-16). People with enough arm strength may use five fingers (or even only three or two fingers) to

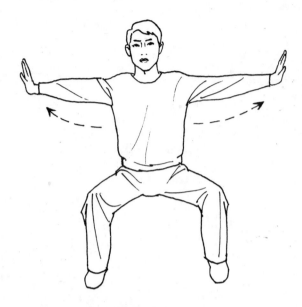

Fig. 2-13 Erlang Immortal Carrying Mount Taishan Exercise

support the body. The exercise may be repeated 9-18 times, according to the physique and age of the performers.

Health Benefits: The exercise can reinforce the strength of fingers and toes,

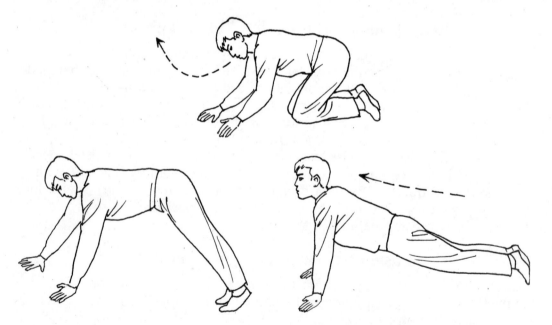

Figs. 2-14, 2-15 and 2-16 Pushing-Up with Dragon's Claws Exercise

strengthen muscles and bones and enrich internal qi.

Healing Applications: The exercise can prevent and treat pains in the neck, shoulder, loins and leg, strengthen the physique and enrich qi for qigong acupressure practice.

Palm-Pushing with Potential Strength

Basic Instructions: In front of a wall or a tree, stand in bow step with one foot behind the other. The back is straight and the palms are put aganist the wall with the five fingers naturally extended or slightly curved like a claw (Fig. 2-17). At the same time, move the Dantian qi to the arms and palms: combine and concentrate mental awareness, qi and strength to push the palms to the wall. The force applied by the palms should be firm but gentle. Then lower your center of gravity and move the palms back and forth naturally (Fig. 2-18). The respiratory movement and the shift of concentrated awareness should keep pace with the movement of arms, and the practioner should stand still and avoid falling down when the body moves back and forth. The force applied by weak practioners should be gentle and increased gradually. Repeat 9-18 times.

Health Benefits: The exercise can reinforce the potential strength of arms and fingers, strengthen the physique and improve the health of the body.

Healing Applications: The exercise can help the functional recovery of injured joints of upper limbs and provide qi for qigong acupressure therapy.

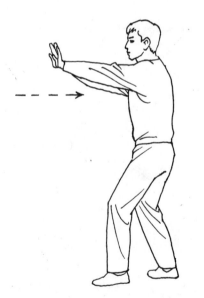

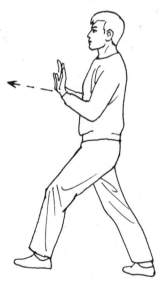

Fig. 2-17 Palm-Pushing with Potential
Strength Exercise

Fig. 2-18 Palm-Pushing with Potential
Strength Exercise

Boy Worshiping the Buddha

Basic Instructions: Assume the Shaolin Post-standing posture. Let the arms hang down freely and the hands gradually raise up from the side of body to the front of the chest with the palms joined together; the inner Laogong (PC 8) points of both hands touch each other; the finger tips reach the shoulder level [Danzhong (RN 17)]; and the elbows are slightly bent to make a square circle, just like a worshiping boy (Fig. 2-19). Concentrate the attention at the inner Laogong point and then move it downward to the lower Dantian. Maintain a natural and smooth respiration. After the stance is maintained for 5-10 minutes, the right arm is pushed out to the right anterolateral side of the body and the left palm is held in front of the abdomen; then the action of both palms is alternately changed and repeated 9-18 times (Figs. 2-20 and 2-21).

Health Benefits: The exercise can produce a sedative effect to adjust the function of brain. It can also generate internal qi.

Healing Applications: The exercise can prevent and treat insomnia, neurasthenia, disturbance of gastrointestinal functions and knee joint diseases.

Closing Posture

After the set of ten postures is finished, use concentrated mental awareness to follow the arms as you raise them up from the side of body to the shoulder level and then turn the palms over and press down to drive the turbid waste qi out of the body.

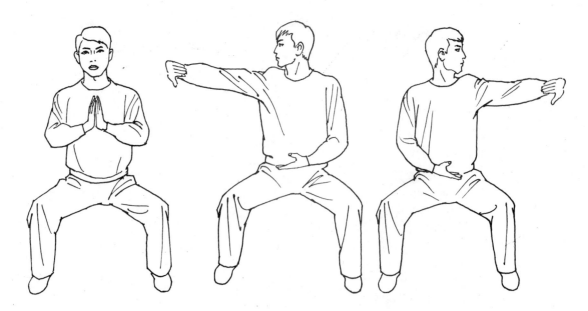

Figs. 2-19, 2-20 and 2-21 Boy Worshiping the Buddha Exercise

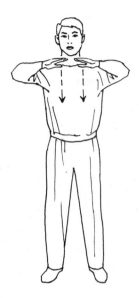

Fig. 2-22 Closing Posture

The body should be relaxed and the respiration should be even and smooth (Fig. 2-22). Repeat 6-8 times.

Notes and Suggestions

1. Practioners may freely choose from these 10 qigong exercises according to their individual needs and ailments. It is best to exercise in the morning after defecation or one hour after breakfast. Your body should be relaxed, your mind and qi harmonious. Physical and mental activities should be coordinated, and respiration should be even and smooth, keeping pace with the physical movements.

2. For beginners, exercises must be performed gently and steadily; the duration and intensity of the exercises should be increased step by step, or else the muscles and bones could be damaged.

3. These exercises should be performed in the morning in a clean and comfortable environment with fresh air. (Breathing fresh air is essential for replenishing vital qi in the body).

4. The sound sleep and nutritious diet can enhance the effect of these physical exercises.

5. Before treating others, qigong acupressure practioners should make sure they have enough medical knowledge and skills regarding qigong acupressure, as well as sufficient qigong practice experience. For self-therapy, the patients should apply qigong acupressure on themselves very gently and slowly; the intensity and duration of stimulation should be gradually increased.

Chapter 3
SUPPLEMENTAL QIGONG ACUPRESSURE THERAPY EXERCISES

Weight Control and Calisthenics

Obesity is usually caused by the internal and external factors. Obesity caused by internal factors is called cerebral or endocrine-dysfunctional adiposity due to hypo-function of the pituitary gland, sexual glands and the thyroid gland. Another type of obesity is due to overeating, lack of physical exercise or bad habits, such as always taking a sitting posture at work. In obese people excess carbohydrates will be pathologically transformed into fat and stored in fatty tissues rather than trans-formed into glycogen, which in normal persons is stored in the liver. Because of the increased thickness of the fatty tissue in abdominal wall, besides reduction of locomotive ability, the patients may suffer from shortness of breath and elevation of blood pressure after physical exertion. Therefore, physical exercise to strengthen muscles of abdominal wall is a good exercise for body weight control and should be performed from the early stages of obesity. But for obesity caused by internal factors, the pathogenic causes should be eliminated.

These exercises for abdominal muscles can produce a massage effect on the internal organs, promote blood circulation and digestive functioning, reduce body weight, and improve functioning of the heart and lungs.

Throughout the entire set of exercises, a natural abdominal respiration with deep inhalation and slow exhalation is maintained; keep your mental awareness concen-trated on following your respiratory movement. The early morning, about 5-6 o'clock (before breakfast), is the best time to do this exercise, but it may also be performed 1-2 hours after meals.

Abdominal Respiration

Basic Instructions: Take a supine posture with arms put on the chest or abdomen and breathe slowly (Fig. 3-1).

Health Benefits: It can strengthen the pectoral muscles and diaphragm.

Duration of Exercise: 3-5 minutes.

Leg-Raising

Basic Instructions: Lie on your back. Keeping them straight and together, as pictured (Fig. 3-2); raise and then lower the legs use natural respiration and

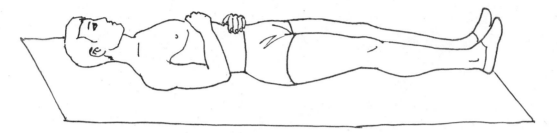

Fig. 3-1 Abdominal Respiration Exercise

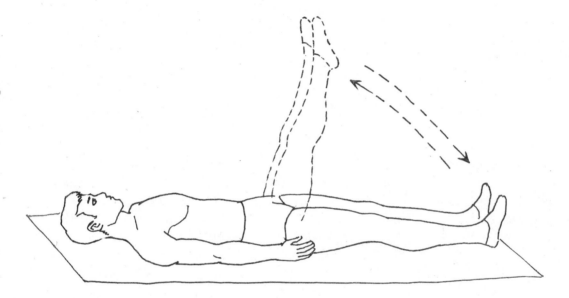

Fig. 3-2 Leg-Raising Exercise

concentrate mental awareness at the Dantian.

Health Benefits: It can strengthen muscles of abdominal wall and buttocks.

Duration of Exercise: 3-5 minutes.

Sit-Ups

Basic Instructions: Do sit-ups with your upper body raised from a supine posture until touching the toes with their fingers (Fig. 3-3). In weak performers it may be done with the nape of the neck embraced by hooked arms and with the legs fixed to the floor by a heavy object or by a person. Respiration should rhythmically follow the movement of body and the mental awareness should be concentrated at Yongquan (KI 1) and middle Dantian.

Health Benefits: It can strengthen the muscles of the abdominal wall.

Duration of Exercise: 3-4 minutes.

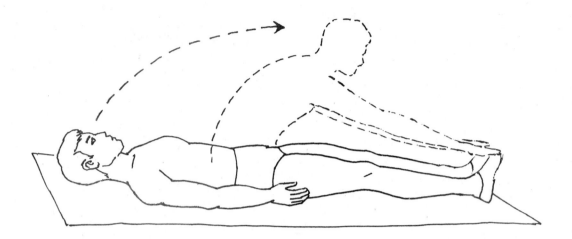

Fig. 3-3 Sit-Up Exercise

Back Stretching

Basic Instructions: Take a supine posture with elbows and knees slightly flexed and heels touching the floor, then lift up and stretch the body using back, abdomen and loin muscles (Fig. 3-4). (The body is supported by the heels, elbows and shoulders.) Respiration should keep pace with body movement; air is inhaled during physical exertion and exhaled during relaxation. Keep your mental awareness concentrated at middle and posterior Dantian.

Health Benefits: It can tonify vital energy, kidney qi and strengthen abdomen, back and loin muscles.

Duration of Exercise: 3-5 minutes.

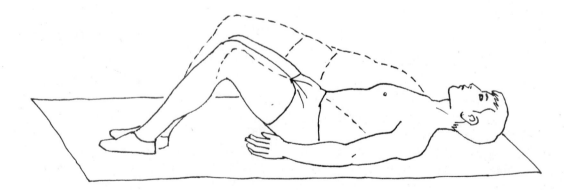

Fig. 3-4 Back Stretching Exercise

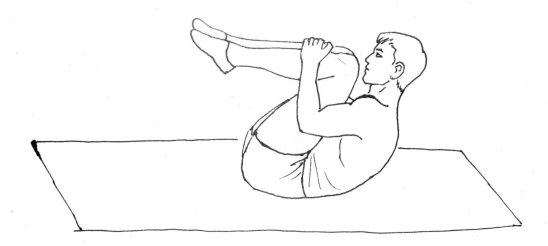

Fig. 3-5 Squeezing the Abdomen Exercise

Squeezing the Abdomen

Basic Instructions: Lie on your back and then lift up and embrace your legs with the arms to squeeze the abdomen (Fig. 3-5).

Health Benefits: It can strengthen the abdominal muscles and stretch the back muscles.

Duration of Exercise: 3-5 minutes.

Cycling

Basic Instructions: Take a supine posture with both legs raised up in the air, and the knees flexed to do cycling (Fig. 3-6). Keep your respiration in pace with your leg movement. Concentrate your mental awareness at the Dantian.

Health Benefits: It can strengthen the ilium muscle and muscles of abdominal wall and pelvic diaphragm.

Duration of Exercise: 3-5 minutes.

Besides the six exercise methods mentioned above, you may do other physical exercises to strengthen abdominal muscles and reduce body weight, such as slow running and swimming.

The duration and times of exercise may be varied according to individuals, ailments and seasons. The whole set of exercises must be performed 1-2 times every day to obtain good results. Alternately, one or several exercises may be practiced to attain a specific healing effect. Beginners should not perform the exercises fast or violently; otherwise, severe pain and soreness of abdominal wall may occur.

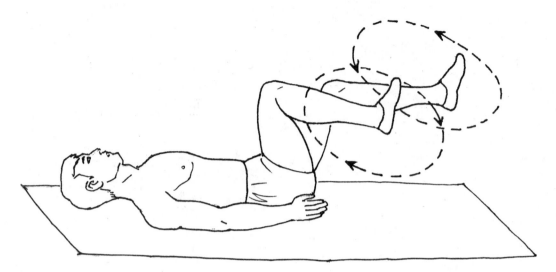

Fig. 3-6 Cycling Exercise

Eight Pieces of Brocade Exercise

This exercise is a traditional eight-segment set modified by adding breathing and mental components to it. It is simple and easy to learn. The intensity and duration may be adjusted according to your physical condition and desired healing effect. You may practise a whole set or few segments (even more repetitions of only one segment) of this set for maintaining health and curing chronic diseases. This is a dynamic exercise and it can benifit both mind and body including (1) strengthening muscles of the four limbs and the chest wall; (2) preventing the development of bad posture, such as kyphosis and scoliosis of spinal column; (3) preventing common chronic diseases, such as cervical scoliosis, leg and lumbago pain, and digestive diseases; and (4) improving brain function, strengthening physique and prolonging life span.

It is best to perform this exercise in the morning and evening in a clean and comfortable environment (such as in park and forest). Practicing the whole set may take 15-30 minutes.

First Segment: Supporting the Heavens

Basic Instructions: Stand with feet parallel, arms hanging down freely, and eyes looking forward. Slowly raise up the arms from both sides of the body, and as the fingers of both hands interlock then turn hands over, palms facing upward, ("supporting the heavens") as you fully extend the arms (Fig. 3-7). Then look at your hands, throw out your chest, hold your abdomen flattened, straighten your back, and then withdraw your arms from both sides back to the starting posture. Repeat the movements several times.

Breathing Instructions: Using concentrated mental awareness to lead the respiration and body movements. During inhalation raise the arms up and turn your palms over to "support the heavens." During exhilation the arms are withdrawn and return to the starting posture. Repeat the movements.

Health Benefits: The exercise adjusts the Sanjiao (Three Energizers) and provides a cardiovascular workout. It can also reduce body weight, prevent and correct kyphosis and scoliosis, strengthen the pectoral muscles, expand the chest cavity, improve respiratory function, facilitate movement of the spinal column and cure cervical spondylosis and constrictive capsulitis.

Second Segment: Shooting a Vulture

Basic Instructions: Stand with the feet shoulder-distance apart, arms hanging down freely, and eyes looking forward. Move your left foot laterally one step to assume a horse-riding posture. Cross the arms at the chest (the left arm inside and the right one outside), and stretch out the fingers. Push the left hand out to the left side until the elbow is fully extended; and make the right hand a clawlike fist to "pull the string of a bow." The tip of right elbow extends laterally and the eyes look at the left hand (Fig. 3-8). The same sequence of actions should be repeated several times on both sides.

Breathing Instructions: Using concentrated mental awareness to lead qi to the pushed out hand. Inhale when the bow is fully drawn and exhale when the full bow is released.

Health Benefits: This exercise is useful to prevent and treat diseases of the neck and shoulder, leg and lumbago pain, chondromalacia of patella and hyperostosis.

Third Segment: Raising up Single Hand

Basic Instructions: Stand with the feet parallel, the arms hanging down freely,

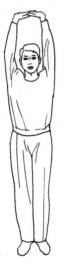

Fig. 3-7

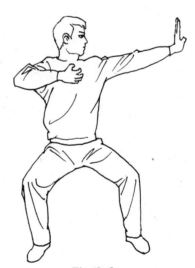

Fig. 3-8

and the eyes looking forward. Raise your left arm up with the palm facing upward. Extend the arm with strength. At the same time, vigorously press your right hand with the palm facing downward and the fingers pointing to the front (Fig. 3-9). Then repeat the sequence with your right hand raised up and your left hand down. Repeat the exercise several times.

Breathing Instructions: Use concentrated mental awareness to lead the qi; coordinate breathe with arm movements. Exhale when arms are fully-extended; inhale when arms are in transition.

Healing Effects: This exercise can adjust the function of the spleen and stomach and it can prevent and treat weakness of the upper limbs and diseases of the digestive system and shoulders.

Fourth Segment: Looking Backward over Shoulder

Basic Instructions: Stand at the attention posture with the neck stretched straight, the arms hanging down freely and the palms touching the thighs. With the chest projected out and the shoulders are squared, slowly rotate your head to the left with your eyes looking backward over your shoulder. Then slowly turn head back to the starting posture. Now, slowly rotate the head to the right in the same manner, returning again to the starting posture. Repeat several times (Fig. 3-10).

Breathing Instructions: Abdominal respiration is maintained through out the exercise. Air is inhaled when you are looking backward; air is exhaled when you turn your head back to the starting posture. The mental attention should be concentrated at the Dantian.

Healing Effects: The exercise is useful to prevent and treat cervical spondylosis and spondiltitis of spinal column.

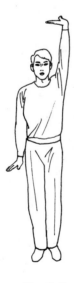

Fig. 3-9

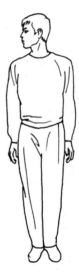

Fig. 3-10

Fifth Segment: Shaking Head and Wagging Tail

Basic Instructions: Using a horse-riding stance, stand with the feet about three feet apart, knees flexed. Put your palms on your knees with the tiger's mouth (part of the hand between the thumb and the forefinger) of hand facing backward to support the straightened trunk. Incline your trunk to the left with the head slightly lowered and shake the head to right side and simultaneously wag the buttocks (tail) to left side (Fig. 3-11). Resume the starting posture. Repeat the movements on the opposite side of the body. This exercise may be performed several times.

Breathing Instructions: Mental awareness is concentrated at the Dantian and a smooth, natural breath is maintained.

Healing Effects: The exercise can improve locomotive function of the waist and knee joints, relieve uneasiness of body and mind, and prevent and treat neurasthenia.

Sixth Segment: Grasping the Feet with Two Hands

Basic Instructions: Stand erect and relaxed with the feet shoulder-distance apart. Bend the upper body forward keeping the knees straightened. The arms hang down and touch the toes with the hands and the eyes look at the hands (Fig. 3-12). Then raise the upper body and bend backward as far as possible, then hold this posture. Place your hands on your lower back with your palms at the Shenshu (BL 23) or Mingmeng (DU 4) points on the back (Fig. 3-13). This exercise may be repeated several times.

Breathing Instructions: The qi is moved in coordination with the shift of concentrated mental attention and the movement of arms. Inhalation begins as you come up from the forward-bending posture and continues into the backward-bending posture. Exhalation begins as you come out of the backward-bending posture and

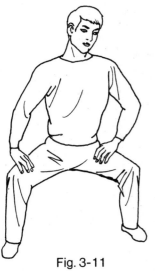

Fig. 3-11

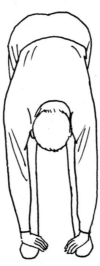

Fig. 3-12

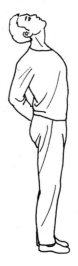

Fig. 3-13

continues as you bend forward. On inhalations transport the qi downward to the posterior Dantian.

Healing Effects: The exercise can strengthen the waist and kidneys, and is also useful to treat lumbago.

Seventh Segment: Opening Eyes Wide with Clenched Fists

Basic Instructions: Take a horse-riding posture and clenched your fists beside the waist, palm-side up. With concentrated mental awareness and twist your left fist slowly forward so the palm-side faces down. At the same time, your right fist is firmly clenched and the left elbow is slowly thrust backward. Your eyes are open wide and staring forward (Fig. 3-14). Then resume the starting posture. Repeat the exercise several times.

Breathing Instructions: Thrust the fists out using concentrated mental awareness. Inhale as fists are thrust forward and back; exhale upon returning to the starting posture. Inhaled air is sent to the middle Dantian to reinforce body strength.

Health Effects: The exercise can strengthen the whole body, especially the limbs. It is also useful to prevent and treat diseases of the neck, shoulder and loins.

Eighth Segment: Standing on Tiptoes

Basic Instructions: Stand erect, with your feet side-by-side and your palms resting against the thighs. Thrust the chest out and straighten your legs as you raise your heels up as high as possible. Using your imagination project the top of head upward (Fig. 3-15). Then lower the heels down to the ground. This exercise may be repeated several times.

Breathing Instructions: The qi is led by the concentrated attention to move in coordination with the movement of body. Inhale as you raise your heels; exhale as

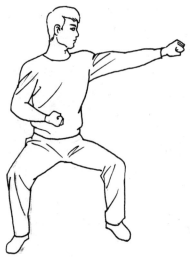

Fig. 3-14

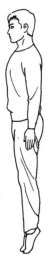

Fig. 3-15

you lower them.

Healing Effects: This exercise can adjust the function of the meridians and it can also lower elevated blood pressure.

Eye Healing Techniques

This exercise program can help improve your eyesight and is effective in treating eye-related ailments.

Starting Postures: Stand with the feet shoulder-distance apart and the palms joined in front of the Dantian. Or take an erect sitting posture with both hands put in front of the chest. Relax the body and quiet the mind. The blood and qi are kept circulating continuously and evenly in the body.

First Technique: With your eyes closed, concentrated mental awareness to move the qi along the Liver Meridian: start from Dadun (LR 1) at the lateral side of big toe and proceed along inner side of the leg into abdomen and then through Qimen (LR 14) along throat and into the eyes. Then, open your eyes and watch a fixed object several meters away and imagin to discharge the turbid (waste) qi from your eyes. This exercise may be repeated several times (Fig. 3-16).

Second Technique: With your eyes closed and mental awareness concentrated at the eyes, move the eye balls up and down in a vertical line, back and forth in a horizontal line, and in a wide circle. Then open your eyes and look forward, to both sides and in a circle. This exercise may be repeated several times (Figs. 3-17, 3-18 and 3-19).

Third Technique: With your eyes closed use your imagination to look at a fixed object (for example, a tree or a flower) a few meters away. Then open your eyes and look at the same object, or look at the object with one eye at a time. This exercise

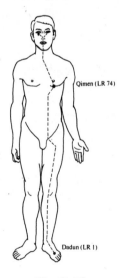

Fig. 3-16

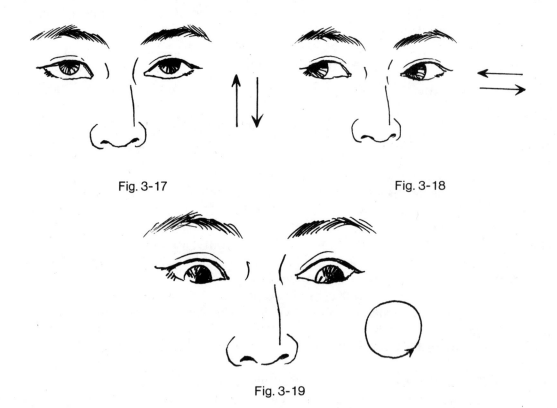

Fig. 3-17   Fig. 3-18

Fig. 3-19

may be repeated several times (Figs. 3-20 and 3-21).

Fourth Technique: Concentrate your mental awareness and qi at the index and middle fingers and massage along the following pathways: (1) from Baihui (DU 20) along the Du Meridian through Shenting (DU 24) to Yintang (EX-HN 3) point (Fig. 3-22); (2) through a circle of acupoints around the eyes from Yintang through

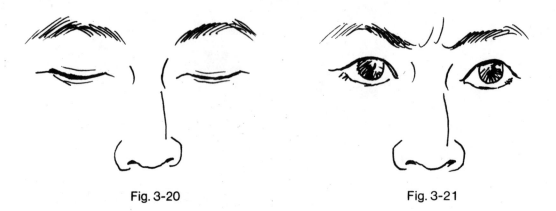

Fig. 3-20   Fig. 3-21

Cuanzhu (BL 2), Yuyao (EX-HN 4, above eyebrow), Sizhukong (SJ 23), Tongziliao (GB 1, at outer canthus), Qiuhou (EX-HN 7), Chengqi (ST 1), Jianming (EX point) to Jingming (BL 1). Massage both clockwise and counterclockwise 7 times each. (Fig. 3-23); (3) from the Baihui through Yintang point to the bilateral eyebrows. After going around both eyes continue through Jingming to Yingxiang (LI 20) and then meet Renzhong (DU 26) and continue through the chest to the Dantian.

Closing Posture: Raise the arms slowly forward and upward to shoulder level; hold the palms facing downward with the finger tips of both hands opposite each other. Press the palms gently downward, finally resting them beside the body or over the Dantian (Fig. 3-24). (In men, the right hand overlaps the left; in women the left hand overlaps the right). Then take a short rest with the eyes closed.

Breathing Instructions: Keep your mind quiet and your breathe smooth and even. The eyes are open when you inhale and closed when you exhale.

Healing Effects: These techniques can adjust the functioning of the brain and eyes, improving eyesight in youths. They can prevent and treat many eye diseases, such as hypopia, myopia, amblyopia, astigmia and hyperopia in aged people. They can also strengthen the brain and treat headache, neurasthenia, insomnia and liver diseases.

Reactions: Some practioners shed tears or feel hotness and relaxation around the eyes in the early stages of practice. Later on, practioners may see red, yellow, green, blue, white or purple spots or rings. These are all qi-sensations, quite normal, and nothing to worry about. If your eyes feel uncomfortable after one to three weeks practice, you can reduce the practice times.

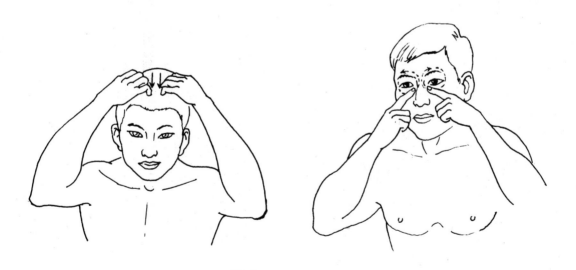

Fig. 3-22   Fig. 3-23

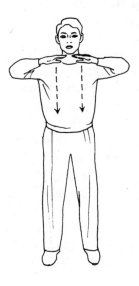

Fig. 3-24

Practice Suggestions: Each technique mentioned above may be repeated 7-21 times; the total eye program should last for 15-30 minutes and be practiced 1-2 times each day.

Chapter 4
BASIC QIGONG ACUPRESSURE
THERAPY TECHNIQUES

Pressing

Techniques

(1) Palm-Pressing: move qi to the hand and concentrate it at the center of the palm; use qi to apply pressure to the injured area or to the acupoints (Fig. 4-1).

(2) Pressing with Two Fingers: move qi to the hand and concentrate it in the extended index and middle fingers. (The other fingers are bent.) Apply pressure to the lesion of a disease or the acupoints (Fig. 4-2).

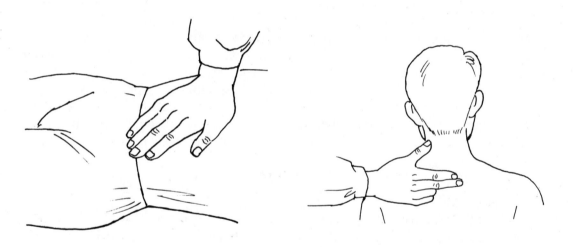

Fig. 4-1 Palm-Pressing Technique   Fig. 4-2 Pressing with Two Fingers Technique

(3) Pressing with Single Finger: move qi to and concentrate at the middle finger (the other fingers are bent) and it is used to apply pressure to the injured area or the acupoints (Fig. 4-3).

(4) Knuckle-Pressing: make a fist; then extend the knuckle of the middle finger out more than the other fingers (Fig. 4-4). Moving qi to the knuckle, use it to apply pressure to the injured area or the acupoints.

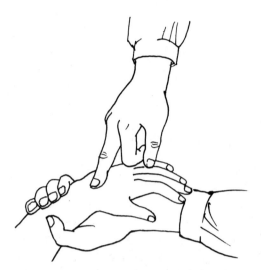

Fig. 4-3 Pressing with Single Finger Technique   Fig. 4-4 Knuckle-Pressing Technique

Notes and Suggestions

This fundamental method of acupressure applies qi and pressure to the diseased area and to the appropriate selected acupoints to treat many common diseases. After you activate your Dantian qi, guide it using concentrated mental awareness, moving through the arm and wrist to the palm, fingers or knuckle; apply pressure and Dantian qi simultaneously to the lesion or acupoints. To produce effective stimulation, pressure and qi should be applied, using the guidance of concentrated mental attention, to the acupoints in a firm but gentle manner to avoid injury to the skin.

Vibrating

Techniques

In clinical practice, the finger, single palm or double palms (Figs. 4-5 and 4-6) are used to apply a vibrating stimulation, along with activated qi, to the injured area or the acupoints.

Notes and Suggestions

Vibrating is an important technique of acupressure used to treat many common diseases. After you concentrate mental attention, move Dantian qi through the arm, elbow and wrist to the palm or finger; apply vibrating stimulation to the lesion of a disease or acupoints, using the palm or finger. Concentrate mental awareness, adjust the breath and move Dantian qi to the palm or finger, and then apply vibrating stimulation gently and slowly according to the therapeutic principle of tonification and reduction. The response of the patient to the treatment should be carefully

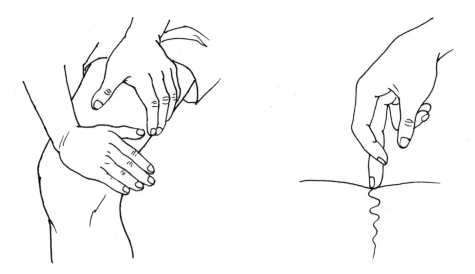

Fig. 4-5 Palm-Vibrating Technique   Fig. 4-6 Finger-Vibrating Technique

watched; adjust the intensity of stimulation as needed.

Knocking

Techniques
Knocking can be divided into the inner side of the fingertip, finger tip and palm methods. The assembled pads of fingers (Fig. 4-7), the assembled tips of the fingers (Fig. 4-8), the central part of palm around the inner Laogong (PC 8) point (Fig. 4-9) or the proximal part (heel) of the palm (Fig. 4-10) may be used to apply knocking stimulation to the injured area or the acupoints.

Notes and Suggestions
Knocking may produce a stimulation over a large area, treating many common diseases. Concentrate mental awareness and guide qi to the hand. Then slowly apply knocking stimulation with appropriate intensity and frequence to the injured area or the acupoints. Dantian qi must be activated and guided to the palm and fingers for applying knocking stimulation with appropriate frequency and intensity to the injured area or acupoints. The knocking stimulation should be not very strong, otherwise the patient's skin may be injured.

Patting

Techniques
Use a slightly concaved palm to pat the body surface over the lesion of a disease (Fig. 4-11). The fingers are slightly bent and separated from each other. With the

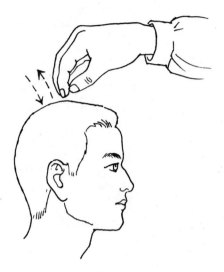

Fig. 4-7 Knocking Technique with the Inner
Side of the Fingertip

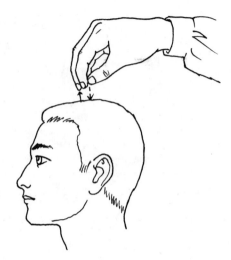

Fig. 4-8 Knocking Technique with Fingertip

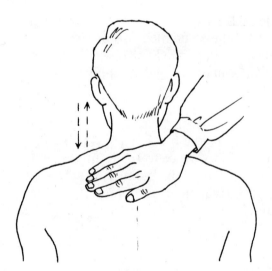

Fig. 4-9 Knocking Technique with Center of
Palm

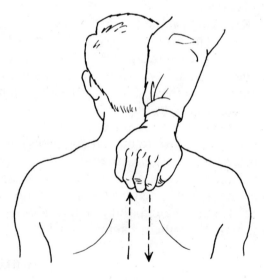

Fig. 4-10 Knocking Technique with Heel of
Palm

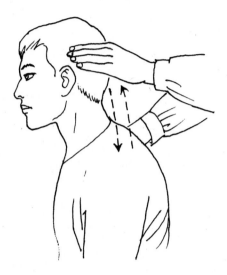

Fig. 4-11 Patting

finger pads and the thenar and hypothenar prominences pat the skin. For areas of the body with thick muscles, use a hollow fist to pat the injured area.

Notes and Suggestions

Patting produces a shaking mechanical stimulation of medium intensity and is usually applied to the limbs, back and loins. Patting can stimulate deep muscles, joints and bones. To apply patting therapy, your shoulders and elbow joints should be relaxed; move your palms up and down rhythmically, patting patients with a frequency of 10-15 times per minute at the beginning of the treatment. Patting frequency and intensity may be gradually increased. Patting can promote the circulation of qi and blood, remove blood stasis in meridians, improve kidney and spleen functioning and strengthen the physique. Heavy patting can stimulate nerves; gentle patting can relax muscles. Before patting therapy, diseases must be correctly diagnosed and the appropriate points should be chosen. The movement of the wrist joint should be flexible and coordinated to produce a springlike feeling. The patting frequency and intensity can be gradually increased to produce heat and relaxation; but it should not be very heavy, otherwise, it may produce adverse effects in patients.

Grasping (Pinching)

Techniques

In this technique the fingers grasp or pinch the muscles and tendons. The skin and muscles at certain places or at some acupoints are grasped or pinched either by

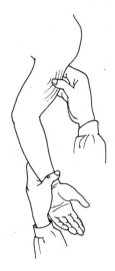

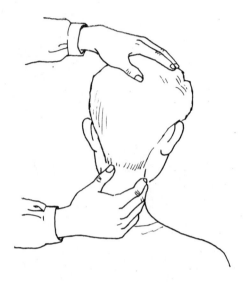

Fig. 4-12 Grasping Exercise   Fig.4-13 Grasping Exercise

the thumb with index and middle finger or with the thumb and the other four fingers to apply an opposing (directed towards each other) pressure with a repeated pinching and relaxing movement (Figs. 4-12 and 4-13).

Notes and Suggestions

Pluck up the local muscle tissue with the thumb and other fingers and then quickly releases them to produce a sore, distending and hot sensation. This technique has strong stimulating effect and is used to treat digestive diseases in children and adults, such as indigestion, abdominal pain, diarrhea, constipation and vomiting. It can be also used to dispel the *wind* and *cold*, promote blood circulation and stop pain. Qigong practioners should move the qi from the Dantian to the hand and then to apply it to the diseased area or acupoints. The pressure should be perpendicularly applied to the skin and muscles, either vertically or horizontally. The tissues avoid persistently pinching muscles without adequate relief and do not use a twisting motion, or the tissues may be injured.

Kneading

Techniques

Kneading is a fundamental technique of acupressure. Fingers, palms, elbows or feet (for the stepping maneuver) are employed to knead the injured area or acupoints. The kneading pressure applied to the body may be either superficial and limited to the skin and muscles or deep enough to reach the bones, joints and internal organs. Kneading pressure may be gradually increased in intensity and held constant for a few seconds and then gradually reduced and released; or it may be applied and

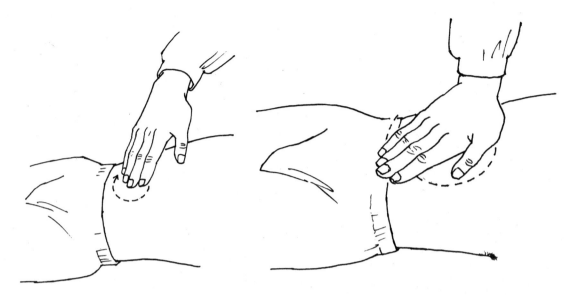

Fig. 4-14 Finger-Kneading Technique   Fig. 4-15 Palm-Kneading Technique

released rhythmically. Either fingers, palms or elbows are used for kneading treatments, depending on the treatment regions.

(1) Finger-kneading: The pad of thumb and/or other fingers (single or multiple) are often used to knead the acupoints or tender spots (*ashi* points) to produce a hot, distending and sore sensation (Fig. 4-14).

(2) Palm-kneading: The central or the heel of palm (single or double) is used to knead the abdomen, back and loins. For the back and loins, kneading may be applied either from the upper part downward or from the lower part upward with a single palm or with the overlapped double palms. The single palm is sufficient to knead the abdomen. Kneading pressure should be rhythmically applied in coordination with the respiratory movement of the patient: kneading and pressing pressure is applied during exhalation and the pressure is releaseed during inhalation (Fig. 4-15).

(3) Elbow-kneading: The tip of elbow is usually used to apply kneading pressure to the lesion of a disease or acupoints in parts of the body with thick muscles, such as the lower back and buttocks or around Huantiao (GB 30) (Fig. 4-16).

Notes and Suggestions

This basic technique of acupressure is often used to treat many common diseases. Concentrated mental awareness must be used to guide Dantian qi to the hand for applying kneading pressure. This will help relax the muscles, eliminate cold evil, relieve spasms and stop pain. As you use the fingers to apply kneading pressure take care to contact the skin slowly and gently; aggressive kneading pressure may damage the patient's skin and soft tissues.

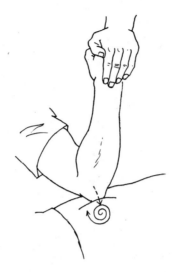

Fig. 4-16 Elbow-Kneading Technique

Push-Rubbing

Techniques

Use your fingers or palms to rub and slide over the body surface or acupoints with a gentle pressure and appropriate strengthen in various directions. Depending on the nature of the disease, the sliding and rubbing speed may be gradually increased from a slow level. The push-rubbing technique can be divided into finger and palm maneuvers.

(1) Push-rubbing with Finger: The pads of fingers are used to rub and slide over the skin or acupoints (Fig. 4-17) on the head, face, back and limbs. Bilateral push-rubbing therapy over Yintang (EX-HN 3) is one example.

(2) Push-rubbing with Palm: The palm is used to rub and slide over the injured area or acupoints (Figs. 4-18 and 4-19) on the chest, abdomen and limbs to improve blood circulation and respiration. The push-rubbing maneuver can be again divided into the gentle and heavy methods.

Notes and Suggestions

This is an important technique in acupressure to treat many diseases. You must concentrate mental awareness and guide Dantian qi through the upper arm, elbow and wrist joints to the palm or fingers and finally to the injured area or acupoints for healing.

Pressure and Frequency of Application: To promote blood circulation, apply the pushing and rubbing pressure gently and quickly with a frequency of 70-80 times per minute; to relax muscles and relieve pain, apply pressure forcibly and slowly with a

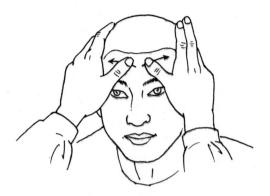

Fig. 4-17 Push-Rubbing Technique with
Finger

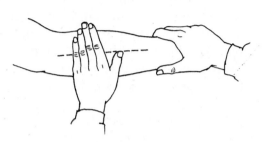

Fig. 4-19 Push-Rubbing Technique with Palm

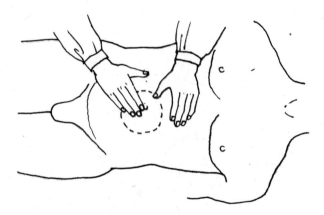

Fig. 4-18 Push-Rubbing Technique with Palm

frequency of 40 times per minute.

Direction of Application

(1) Centrifugal: Apply pressure from the body trunk to the distal ends of limbs to promote circulation of qi and blood.

(2) Centripetal: Apply pressure from the distal ends of limbs to the body trunk to remove blood stasis and eliminate pathogenic evils.

(3) Radiating: Apply pressure radiating out from the center of injured area or acupoint to resolve swelling and lump.

(4) Inward: Apply pressure starting from the peripheral areas of a injured area or acupoint and work towards the center. This promotes blood circulation and resolves swelling.

(5) Back and forth: Apply pressure backward and forward: for example, centrifugal pushing pressure may be applied forward 3 times and backward for 1 time to adjust qi and blood; and centripetal pushing pressure may be applied forward 3 times and backward 1 time to relieve blood stasis. The 1 forward and 3 backward pushing in a centrifugal direction tonifies qi; 1 forward and 3 backward pushing in a centripetal direction disperses qi. The appropriate type of push-rubbing maneuver depends on your diagnosis of the patient's condition; effective treatment of disease depends on the skillful application of the maneuver.

Rolling

Techniques

After qi is activated and guided to the hand, use the lateral hypothenar border of

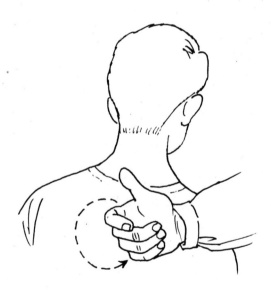

Fig. 4-20 Rolling over Back Technique

your hollow fist to repeatedly roll back and forth over the injured area or acupoints using a rhythmic and flexible wrist movement (Fig. 4-20).

Notes and Suggestions

Use the lateral border of your hand on the lesion of a disease or acupoints and apply a continuous rolling pressure with the 3rd, 4th and 5th metacarpal bones and the forearm, maintaining flexible wrist movement. During treatment, qi is activated and guided to the outer Laogong (EX-point) point producing a hot and relaxing sensation in patients.

The dorsum of rolling hand must be closely adhered to the patient's skin and rolling pressure must be continuously and evenly applied to the acupoints, joints and muscles along the meridians. Rolling pressure is usually applied over a large area of the body surface and deep into the muscles. Avoid any jerking, hitting or rubbing movement of the hand that could cause injury to the skin and underlying tissues.

This is an important acupressure technique; it is usually used for health maintenance in critical and weak patients and also for treatment of chronic internal diseases.

Chapter 5
LOCATION AND HEALING APPLICATIONS OF COMMON ACUPOINTS AND CLINICAL FORMULAE

To obtain better therapeutic results using qigong acupressure therapy, the qigong practioners should know the location and indications of acupoints of the 14 meridians and understand the time-related circulation of qi and blood through the meridians.

Concept of Meridians and Acupoints

Through the clinical practice to struggle against the diseases of human beings for more than two thousand years, Chinese physicians discovered the close functional connection between different parts of human body: for example, the stimulation at Hegu (LI 4) may affect the function of the head, face, nose and throat; stimulation at Neiguan (PC 6) of the forearm may affect functioning of the heart and blood vessels; and stimulation at Zusanli (ST 36) on the anterior surface of the leg may affect functioning of the stomach and intestines. In traditional Chinese medicine, the anatomical energetic channels of the human body are known as *jingluo* (meridians): *Jings* are the main trunks, deeply situated in the interior part of the body; and the *luos* are the superficial fine branches that link the *jings*. Along the meridians there are many spots, called *jingxue* (acupoints), which when mechanically and thermally stimulated produce strong responses and therapeutic effects in the body. The *jingluo* (meridian) system is composed of the Du Meridian, the Ren Meridian and meridians of the twelve organs, including the six Zang Organs: heart, liver, spleen, lungs, kidney and pericarium and the six Fu Organs: gallbladder, stomach, large intestine, small intestine, urinary bladder and Sanjiao (Three Energizers). The organ meridians are named after their related organs: for example, the meridian connected with the heart organ is called the Heart Meridian; and the meridian related to the stomach is called the Stomach Meridian. The meridians that pass through upper limbs are called Hand Meridians and those that pass through lower limbs are called Foot Meridians. The meridians of the six Zang Organs always pass through the medial surface of the four limbs are called Yin Meridians; and those of the six Fu Organs always pass through the lateral surface of the limbs are called Yang Meridians. The Yin Meridians may be further divided into the Shaoyin, Jueyin and Taiyin Meridians and they are arranged regularly along the radial, middle or ulnar line on the medial surface of the arms or along the anterior, middle or posterior line on the medial surface of the legs. The correspondent Yang Meridians on the lateral surface of the four limbs are the Yangming, Shaoyang and Taiyang meridians. The Taiyin and Yangming, Jueyin and Shaoyang as well as the Shaoyin and Taiyang meridians are closely related pairs. The Ren and Du meridians originate from the same organ, *Baogong* (uterus) but they travel different courses after they emerge from perineum. As a Yin Meridian, the Ren Meridian is linked with the other six Yin Meridians as it travels upward along the anterior midline; and as a Yang Meridian, the Du Meridian is linked with all six Yang Meridians as it travels upward along the posterior midline. Therefore, they are closely related with the twelve organs and their correlated meridians. (Figs. 5-1, 2, 3)

Courses and Acupoints of the 14 Meridians

Lung Meridian of Hand-Taiyin

Course: Lateral chest wall—› radial line of medial surface of upper limbs—› radial surface of thumbs

Acupoints: Zhongfu (LU 1), Chize (LU 5), Lieque (LU 7) and Shaoshang (LU 11)

Healing Applications: Chest, lungs and throat diseases

Pericardium Meridian of Hand-Jueyin

Course: Lateral side of nipples—› chest—› middle line of medial surface of upper limbs—› tip of middle fingers

Acupoints: Tianchi (PC 1), Jianshi (PC 5), Neiguan (PC 6), Daling (PC 7) and Zhongchong (PC 9)

Healing Applications: Chest, heart and stomach diseases

Heart Meridian of Hand-Shaoyin

Course: Axillary pit—› ulnar line of medial surface of the upper limbs—›radial surface of little fingers

Acupoints: Jiquan (HT 1), Shenmen (HT 7), Shaohai (HT 3) and Shaochong (HT 9)

Healing Applications: Brain, heart, and mental diseases

Large Intestine Meridian of Hand-Yangming

Course: Radial surface of index fingers—› radial line of lateral surface of upper limbs—› anterior surface of shoulders—› neck—› teeth of lower jaw—› paranasal region

Acupoints: Shangyang (LI 1), Hegu (LI 4), Quze (LI 11), Jianyu (LI 15) and Yingxiang (LI 20)

Healing Applications: Head, face, eyes, nose, oral cavity, teeth, throat and febrile diseases

Sanjiao Meridian of Hand-Shaoyang

Course: Ulnar surface of ring fingers—> middle line of lateral surface of upper limbs—> upper surface of shoulder—> neck—> postauricular region—> lateral end of eyebrow

Acupoints: Guanchong (SJ 1), Zhongzhu (SJ 3), Waiguan (SJ 5), Zhigou (SJ 6), Yifeng (SJ 17) and Sizhukong (SJ 23)

Healing Applications: Temporal area, eyes, ears, throat, chest and febrile diseases

Small Intestine Meridian of Hand-Taiyang

Course: Ulnar surface of little fingers—> ulnar line of lateral surface of upper limbs—> scapula—> neck—> region below eyes—> preauricular region

Acupoints: Shaoze (SI 1), Tianzong (SI 11), Jianwaishu (SJ 14) and Tinggong (SI 19)

Healing Applications: Head, neck, eyes, throat, mental and febrile diseases

Stomach Meridian of Foot-Yangming

Course: Area below eyes—> teeth of upper jaw—> face—> anterior surface of neck —> chest and abdomen—> anterior line of lateral surface of lower limbs—> lateral surface of 2nd toe

Acupoints: Chengqi (ST 1), Dicang (ST 4), Jiache (ST 6), Xiaguan (ST 7), Tianshu (ST 25), Zusanli (ST 36) and Lidui (ST 45)

Healing Applications: Head, face, oral cavity, teeth, throat, stomach, intestines, mental and febrile diseases

Gallbladder Meridian of Foot-Shaoyang

Course: Outer canthus of eye—> top of head—> lateral area of top of head—> nape—> chest—> lateral surface of waist —> lateral surface of lower limbs—> lateral surface of fourth toe

Acupoints: Fengchi (GB 20), Jianjing (GB 21), Huantiao (GB 30), Yanglingquan (GB 34), Tinghui (GB 2), Yangbai (GB 14) and Zuqiaoyin (GB 44)

Healing Applications: Temporal area, eyes, ears, liver, ribs, gallbladder and febrile diseases

Urinary Bladder Meridian of Foot-Taiyang

Course: Inner canthus of eyes—> top of head—> neck—> bilateral area of spinal column—> posterior surface of lower limbs—> lateral malleolus—> lateral surface of little toes

Acupoints: Jingming (BL 1), Cuanzhu (BL 2), Feishu (BL 13), Ganshu (BL 18), Danshu (BL 19), Pishu (BL 20), Kunlun (BL 60) and Zhiyin (BL 67)

Healing Applications: Top of head, eyes, loins and back, mental and febrile diseases

Spleen Meridian of Foot-Taiyin

Course: Medial surface of big toes—› anterior line of medial surface of legs—› middle line of medial surface of legs—› anterior line of medial surface of thighs—› lateral surface of abdomen and chest

Acupoints: Yinbai (SP 1), Sanyinjiao (SP 6), Yinlingquan (SP 9) and Xuehai (SP 10)

Healing Applications: Abdomen, urogenital system, stomach, intestines and endocrine system diseases

Liver Meridian of Foot-Jueyin

Course: Lateral surface of big toes—› anterior line of medial surface of legs—› middle line of medial surface of legs—› middle line of medial surface of thighs—› external genital organ—› flank region

Acupoints: Dadun (LR 1), Xingjian (LR 2), Taichong (LR 3), Zhangmen (LR 13) and Qimen (LR 14)

Healing Applications: Abdomen, urogenital system, liver and gallbladder diseases

Kidney Meridian of Foot-Shaoyin

Course: Center of soles—› posterior line of medial surface of lower limbs—› abdomen (near anterior midline)—› chest (near anterior midline)

Acupoints: Yongquan (KI 1), Taixi (KI 3), Zhaohai (KI 6), Fuliu (KI 7) and Shufu (KI 27)

Healing Applications: Abdomen, urogenital system, lungs and throat diseases

Ren Meridian

Course: Perineum—› anterior midline of abdomen and chest—›neck—› midpoint of lower lip

Acupoints: Huiyin (RN 1), Guanyuan (RN 4), Qihai (RN 6), Zhongwan (RN 12), Danzhong (RN 17), Tiantu (RN 22) and Chengjiang (RN 24)

Healing Applications: Throat, chest, lungs, stomach, intestines, urogenital and endocrinal system diseases

Du Meridian

Course: Coccyx—› spinal column—› neck—› midline of head—› forehead—› nose—› midpoint of upper lip

Acupoints: Changqiang (DU 1), Mingmen (DU 4), Dazhui (DU 14), Baihui (DU 20), Shangxing (DU 23), Renzhong (DU 26) and Yinjiao (DU 28)

Healing Applications: Head, face, throat, chest, urogenital and endocrinal system and mental diseases

Common Acupoints for Qigong Acupressure

Besides the course and healing applications of the 14 meridians, practioners

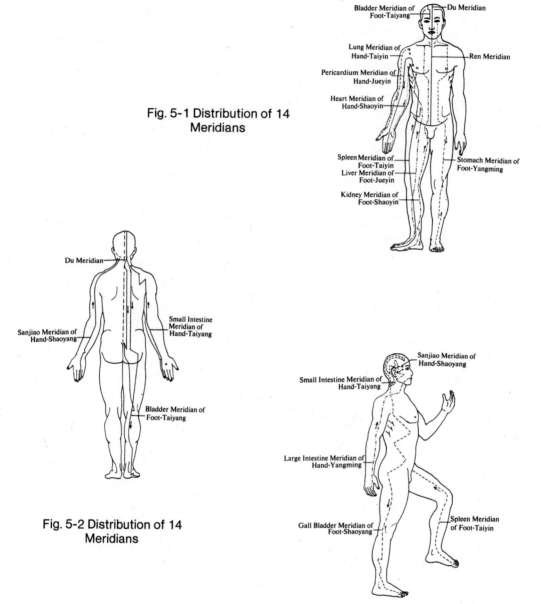

Fig. 5-1 Distribution of 14
Meridians

Bladder Meridian of
Foot-Taiyang
Du Meridian

Lung Meridian of
Hand-Taiyin
Ren Meridian

Pericardium Meridian of
Hand-Jueyin

Heart Meridian of
Hand-Shaoyin

Spleen Meridian of
Foot-Taiyin
Stomach Meridian of
Foot-Yangming
Liver Meridian of
Foot-Jueyin

Kidney Meridian of
Foot-Shaoyin

Du Meridian

Small Intestine
Meridian of
Hand-Taiyang

Sanjiao Meridian of
Hand-Shaoyang

Bladder Meridian of
Foot-Taiyang

Fig. 5-2 Distribution of 14
Meridians

Sanjiao Meridian of
Hand-Shaoyang

Small Intestine Meridian of
Hand-Taiyang

Large Intestine Meridian of
Hand-Yangming

Gall Bladder Meridian of
Foot-Shaoyang

Spleen Meridian
of Foot-Taiyin

Fig. 5-3 Distribution of 14
Meridians

should also remember the location of common acupoints for clinical practice.

Head, Face, Neck and Nape Regions (Figs. 5-4, 5-5 and 5-6)

Shenting (DU 24): Directly above nose and 0.5 cun above anterior hair line

Yintang (EX-HN 3): At the midpoint between bilateral eyebrows and directly above apex of nose

Yuyao (EX-HN 4): At the midpoint of eyebrows

Chengqi (ST 1): 0.7 cun below eyes

Shuigou (DU 26): At the junction of upper and middle one-third of philtrum of upper lip

Yingxiang (LI 20): 0.5 cun beside nostril

Chengjiang (RN 24): In the depression below the midpoint of lower lip

Baihui (DU 20): 5 cun above anterior hair line and at midpoint between bilateral auricular apices

Fengchi (GB 20): On nape and below occipital bone, in the depression lateral to the tendon of trapezius muscle and on the same level of Fengfu (DU 16)

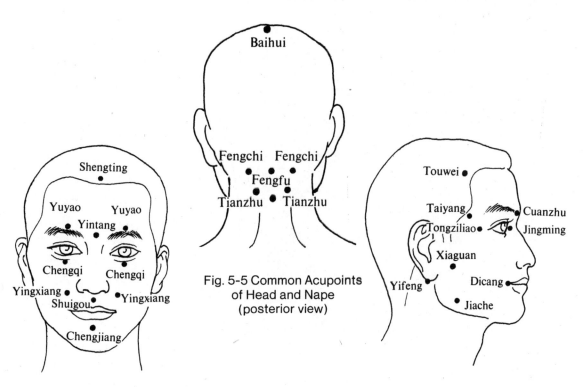

Fig. 5-5 Common Acupoints
of Head and Nape
(posterior view)

Fig. 5-4 Common Acupoints
of the Face (anterior view)

Fig. 5-6 Common Acupoints
of Head and Face
(lateral view)

Fengfu (DU 16): Below occipital bone and 1 cun above posterior hair line

Tianzhu (BL 10): On the posterior hair line (between 1st and 2nd cervical vertebrae) and in the depression beside the tendon of trapezius muscle

Touwei (ST 8): At the bilateral corner of forehead and 0.5 cun above anterior hair line, and 4.5 cun lateral to Shenting (DU 24)

Taiyang (EX-HN 5): In a depression 1 finger-width lateral and below lateral end of eyebrows

Cuanzhu (BL 2): In a depression at the medial end of eyebrows

Jingming (BL 1): In a depression 0.1 cun medial to the inner canthus of eyes

Tongziliao (GB 1): 0.5 cun behind the outer canthus of eyes

Xiaguan (ST 7): In a depression below zygomatic arch and in front of anterior auricular artery

Yifeng (SJ 17): In a depression 0.5 cun behind the ear lobes

Jiache (ST 6): 1 cun below ears and in the masseter muscle on the mandibular angle

Dicang (ST 4): 0.4 cun lateral to the mouth angle

Shoulder, Back, Lumbar and Hip Regions (Fig. 5-7)

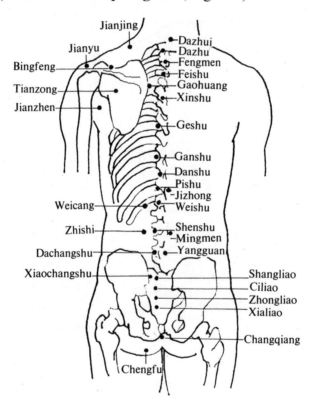

Fig. 5-7 Common Acupoints on the Shoulder, Back, Loins and Buttocks

Jianjing (GB 21): Above supraclavicular fossa, in front of scapula and slightly anterior to the midpoint between Dazhui (DU 14) and Jianyu (LI 15)

Dazhui (DU 14): Below the spinous process of 7th cervical vertebra

Dazhu (BL 11): On the nape, below the 1st thoracic vertebra and 1.5 cun lateral to the posterior midline

Jianyu (LI 15): In a cleft between two bones on the acromion of shoulder with a depression when the arm is raised up.

Fengmen (BL 12): Below the second thoracic vertebra and 1.5 cun lateral to the posterior midline

Bingfeng (SI 12): At the lateral corner of suprascapular fossa [2 cun lateral to Quyuan (SI 13)]

Feishu (BL 13): Below the 3rd thoracic vertebra and 1.5 cun lateral to the posterior midline

Gaohuang (BL 43): Below the 4th thoracic vertebra and 3 cun lateral to the posterior midline

Jianzhen (SI 9): Between the two bones behind the acromion of shoulder and 1 cun above the posterior end of axillary crease

Xinshu (BL 15): Below the 5th thoracic vertebra and 1.5 cun lateral to the posterior midline

Tianzong (SI 11): In a depression below the scapular spine, directly below Bingfen (SI 12) and on the level of 4th thoracic vertebra

Geshu (BL 17): Below the 7th thoracic vertebra and 1.5 cun lateral to the posterior midline

Ganshu (BL 18): Below the 9th thoracic vertebra and 1.5 cun lateral to the posterior midline

Danshu (BL 19): Below the 10th thoracic vertebra and 1.5 cun lateral to the posterior midline

Pishu (BL 20): Below the 11th thoracic vertebra and 1.5 cun lateral to the posterior midline

Jizhong (DU 6): Below the 11th thoracic vertebra

Weicang (BL 50): Below the 12th thoracic vertebra and 3 cun lateral to the posterior midline

Weishu (BL 21): Below the 12th thoracic vertebra and 1.5 cun lateral to the posterior midline

Zhishi (BL 52): Below the 2nd lumbar vertebra and 3 cun lateral to the posterior midline on the level of Shenshu (BL 23)

Shenshu (BL 23): Below the 2nd lumbar vertebra and 1.5 cun lateral to the posterior midline

Mingmen (DU 4): Below the 2nd lumbar vertebra

Dachangshu (BL 25): Below the 4th lumbar vertebra and 1.5 cun lateral to the posterior midline

Yangguan (DU 3): Below the 4th lumbar vertebra

Xiaochangshu (BL 27): Below the 1st sacral vertebra and 1.5 cun lateral to the posterior midline

Shangliao (BL 30): Beside the 1st sacral vertebra and in the 1st sacral foramen

Ciliao (BL 31): Beside the 2nd sacral vertebra and in the 2nd sacral foramen

Zhongliao (BL 32): Beside the 3rd sacral vertebra and in the 3rd sacral foramen

Xialiao (BL 33): Beside the 4th sacral vertebra and in the 4th sacral foramen

Changqiang (DU 1): 0.5 cun below the tip of coccyx

Chengfu (BL 36): At the midpoint of inferior gluteal crease

Chest and Abdomen Regions (Fig. 5-8)

Tiantu (RN 22): In the suprasternal fossa (with the chin up for insertion of needle)

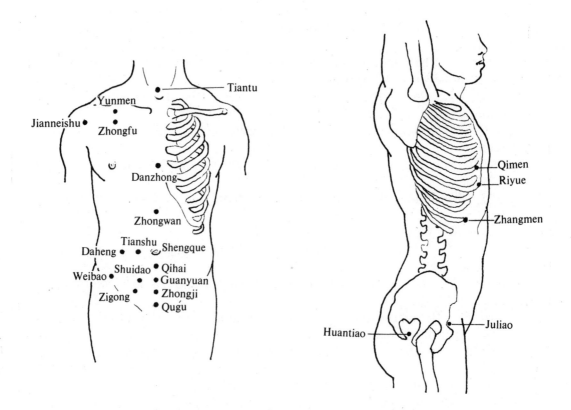

Fig. 5-8 Common Acupoints on the Chest and Abdomen

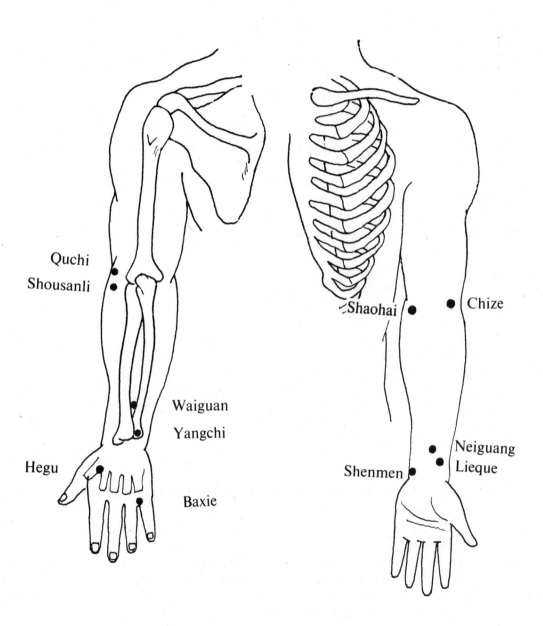

Fig. 5-9 Common Acupoints on the Upper Limbs

Yunmen (LU 2): Below the clavicle and the coracoid process and medial to the head of humerus, 6 cun lateral to the anterior midline

Zhongfu (LU 1): Above the breast, in the 3rd intercostal space and 1 cun below Yunmen (LU 2)

Jianneishu (SI 15): On the anterior border of deltoid muscle and opposite to Jianwaishu (SI 14)

Danzhong (RN 17): On the anterior midline and at the midpoint between bilateral nipples

Qimen (LR 14): Two ribs directly below nipples and 4 cun lateral to the anterior midline

Riyue (GB 24): 0.5 cun below Qimen (LR 14)

Zhangmen (LR 13): In the hypochondriac region and at the terminal end of 11th rib

Juliao (GB 29): At the midpoint between the anterosuperior iliac spine and the prominence of great trochanter

Huantiao (GB 30): At the junction of the middle and lateral, one-third between the great trochanter and sacral hiatus (when a person is in a lateral recumbent posture with the thigh flexed)

Zhongwan (RN 12): 4 cun above umbilicus

Daheng (SP 15): 4 cun lateral to umbilicus

Tianshu (ST 25): 2 cun lateral to umbilicus

Shenque (RN 8): In the pit of umbilicus

Qihai (RN 6): 1.5 cun below umbilicus

Weibao (EX-point): In the inguinal region

Guanyuan (RN 4): 3 cun below umbilicus

Shuidao (ST 28): 3 cun below umbilicus and 2 cun lateral to the anterior midline

Zigong (EX-CA 1): 3 cun lateral to Zhongji (RN 3)

Zhongji (RN 3): 4 cun below umbilicus

Qugu (RN 2): 5 cun below umbilicus

Upper Limbs (Fig. 5-9)

Shaohai (HT 3): About 0.5 cun distal to medial epicondyle on the medial surface of humerus, as the elbow is flexed

Chize (LU 5): In a depression in the cubital crease lateral to the tendon of brachial biceps muscle

Neiguan (PC 6): 2 cun proximal to the carpal crease between two tendons

Lieque (LU 7): On the radial side of the forearm, 1.5 cun proximal to the carpal crease and at a point where the tip of index finger may reach when the tiger's mouth of both hands crisscross with each other

Shenmen (HT 7): In a depression at the ulnar end of carpal crease and proximal to a bony prominence

Quchi (LI 11): In a depression at the lateral end of cubital crease

Shousanli (LI 10): 2 cun distal to Quchi (LI 11)

Waiguan (SJ 5): 2 cun proximal to the dorsal carpal crease and between two bones

Yangchi (SI 4): In a depression on the dorsal carpal crease directly proximal to the 4th metacarpal bone

Hegu (LI 4): On the dorsum of hand at the midpoint of the radial side of 2nd metacarpal bone

Baxie (EX-UE 9): Four points on each hand, at the margin of webs between neighbouring fingers

Lower Limbs (Figs. 5-10, 5-11, 5-12 and 5-13)

Biguan (ST 31): Above Futu (ST 32) point on the level of perineum

Futu (ST 32): 6 cun above patella and on the prominent part of muscles of thigh

Fengshi (GB 31): 7 cun above knee joint at a point where the tip of middle finger may reach when the arm freely hangs down

Heding (EX-LE 2): 1 cun directly above patella

Xiyan (EX-LE 5): In the depressions below patella and beside tendon

Yanglingquan (GB 34): 2 cun below knee joint and in a depression in front of the head of fibula

Yinlingquan (SP 9): 2 cun below knee joint, in a depression below the medial condyle of tibia, and opposite Yanglingquan (GB 34)

Zusanli (ST 36): 3 cun below Xiyan (EX-LE 5) and 1 cun beside tibial crest

Sanyinjiao (SP 6): 3 cun directly above the medial malleolus

Jiexi (ST 41): In the dorsal crease between the instep and leg directly above the 2nd metatarsal bone

Weizhong (BL 40): At the center of popliteal fossa

Chengshan (BL 57): In the cleft of calf muscles

Xuanzhong (GB 39): 3 cun above lateral malleolus in front of the fibula

Kunlun (BL 60): In a depression above heel and 0.5 cun behind lateral malleolus

Taixi (KI 3): Above heel and 0.5 cun behind medial malleolus

Yongquan (KI 1): At the center of sole and at the junction between anterior two-fifths and posterior three-fifths of foot

Anterior and Posterior Midlines (Fig. 5-14)

Qigong Acupressure and the Three Symbols of Yin and Yang (Fig. 5-15)

The concept of three symbols of yin and yang was derived from ancient Chinese dialectic philosophy to objectively explain the phenomena, events and nature of the universe, which were believed to be constantly and dynamically changing while maintaining a balance between opposites. As shown in the chart, the upper symbol is a circle of pure yang to represent the heavens, the lower one

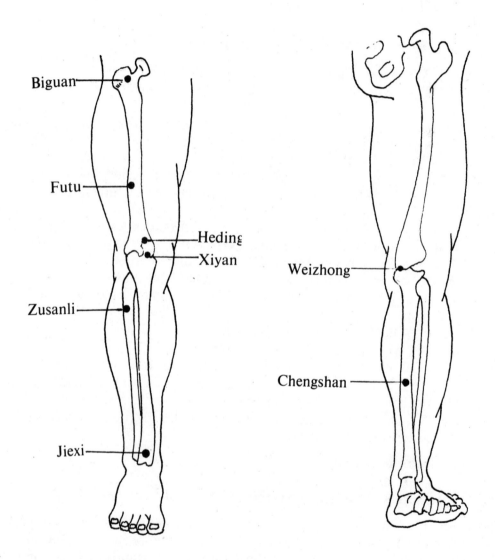

Figs. 5-10 and 5-11 Common Acupoints on the Lower Limbs

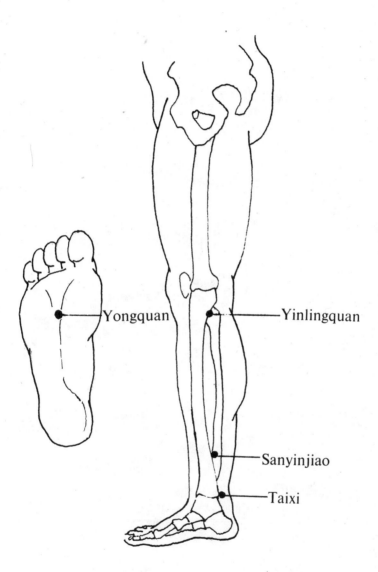

Fig. 5-12 Common Acupoints on the Lower Limb

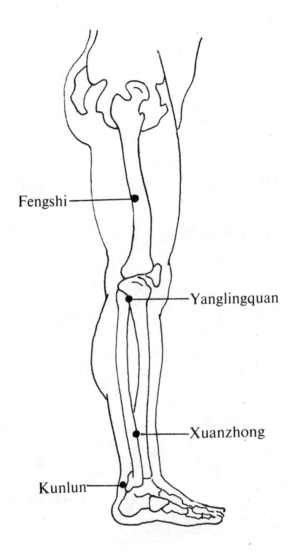

Fig. 5-13 Common Acupoints on the Lower Limb

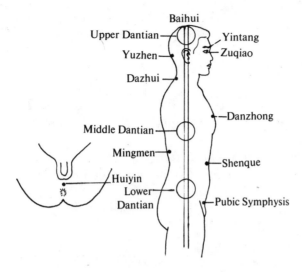

Fig. 5-14 Dantians and Common Acupoints on Midlines

is a circle of pure yin to represent the earth, and the middle one is a mixed circle of yin and yang to represent mankind. In qigong acupressure therapy, the upper circle is the upper Dantian, the lower one is the lower Dantian, and the middle one is the middle Dantian in human body. The qi for qigong acupressure therapy is activated and modulated in those Dantians and then it is guided to the hands

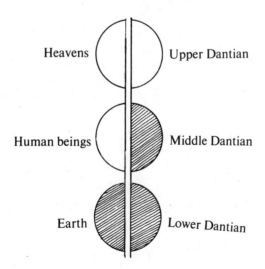

Fig. 5-15 Qigong Acupressure and Three Symbols of Yin and Yang

and used for healing patients.

Acupoint Formulae for Qigong Acupressure Therapy

Diseases of Nervous System

Frontal Headache
Principal Acupoints: Yintang (EX-HN 3), Qianding (DU 21) and Touwei (ST 8);
Supplemental Acupoints: Shangxing (DU 23) and Waiguan (SJ 5)

Parietal Headaches
Principal Acupoints: Baihui (DU 20), Qianding (DU 21) and Houding (DU 19);
Supplemental Acupoints: Hegu (LI 4) and Fengchi (GB 20)

Occipital Headaches
Principal Acupoints: Fengchi (GB 20), Houding (DU 19) and Tianzhu (BL 10);
Supplemental Acupoints: Yuzhen (BL 9) and Hegu (LI 4)

Temporal Headaches
Principal Acupoints: Taiyang (EX-HN 5), Touwei (ST 8) and Hegu (LI 4);
Supplemental Acupoints: Fengchi (GB 20) and Waiguan (SJ 5)

Dizziness and Sleepiness
Principal Acupoints: Hegu (LI 4), Shaoshang (LU 11) and Fengchi (GB 20);
Supplemental Acupoints: Baihui (DU 20) and Chize (LU 5)

Anemia with Dizziness
Principal Acupoints: Taiyang (EX-HN 5), Jiexi (ST 41) and Fenglong (ST 40);
Supplemental Acupoints: Hegu (LI 4) and Zusanli (ST 36)

Neurosthenia with Insomnia
Principal Acupoints: Shenmen (HT 7), Waiguan (SJ 5) and Shaochong (HT 9);
Supplemental Acupoints: Hegu (LI 4) and Zusanli (ST 36)

Insomnia Due to Digestive Diseases
Principal Acupoints: Zusanli (ST 36), Zhongwan (RN 12) and Guanyuan
  (RN 4);
Supplemental Acupoints: Neiguan (PC 6), Qihai (RN 6) and Dachangshu
  (BL 25)

Insomnia Due to Coronary Heart Disease
Principal Acupoints: Neiguan (PC 6), Zusanli (ST 36) and Laogong (PC 8);
Supplemental Acupoints: Shenmen (HT 7) and Xinshu (BL 15)

Insomnia Due to Endocrinal Diseases
Principal Acupoints: Hegu (LI 4), Quchi (LI 11) and Feishu (BL 13);
Supplemental Acupoints: Sanyinjiao (SP 6) and Zusanli (ST 36)

Diseases of Respiratory System

Cough
Principal Acupoints: Taiyuan (LU 9) and Yunmen (LU 2);
Supplemental Acupoints: Hegu (LI 4) and Chize (LU 5)

Cough with Phlegm
Principal Acupoints: Feishu (BL 13), Tiantu (RN 22) and Fenglong (ST 40);
Supplemental Acupoints: Hegu (LI 4) and Chize (LU 5)
Chronic Cough and Asthma
Principal Acupoints: Taiyuan (LU 9), Yunmen (LU 2) and Feishu (BL 13);
Supplemental Acupoints: Chize (LU 5) and Hegu (LI 4)
Asthma
Principal Acupoints: Tiantu (RN 22), Hegu (LI 4) and Danzhong (RN 17);
Supplemental Acupoints: Houxi (SI 3) and Zusanli (ST 36)
Anterior Chest Pain
Principal Acupoints: Neiguan (PC 6), Quchi (LI 11) and Daling (PC 7);
Supplemental Acupoints: Danzhong (RN 17) and Hegu (LI 4)
Posterior Chest Pain
Principal Acupoints: Waiguan (SJ 5), Tianzong (SI 11) and Zhigou (SJ 6);
Supplemental Acupoints: Weizhong (BL 40) and Zhangmen (LR 13)

Symptoms of Digestive System

Febrile Diseases
Principal Acupoints: Jinjin (EX-HN 12) and Yuye (EX-HN 13);
Supplemental Acupoints: Neiguan (PC 6) and Zusanli (ST 36)
Chest Diseases
Principal Acupoints: Hegu (LI 4), Shaoshang (LU 11) and Zusanli (ST 36);
Supplemental Acupoints: Danzhong (RN 17) and Chize (LU 5)
Stomach and Intestine Diseases
Principal Acupoints: Zusanli (ST 36), Neiguan (PC 6) and Zhongwan (RN 12);
Supplemental Acupoints: Guanyuan (RN 4) and Weishu (BL 21)
Inner-Ear Diseases
Principal Acupoints: Fengchi (GB 20), Yifeng (SJ 17) and Tianzhu (BL 10);
Supplemental Acupoints: Hegu (LI 4) and Chize (LU 5)
Gynaecological Diseases
Principal Acupoints: Sanyinjiao (SP 6), Hegu (LI 4) and Xuehai (SP 10);
Supplemental Acupoints: Qihai (RN 6) and Zusanli (ST 36)
Poor Appetite
Principal Acupoints: Zusanli (ST 36), Quchi (LI 11) and Zhigou (SJ 6);
Supplemental Acupoints: Zhongwan (RN 12) and Neiguan (PC 6)
Stomachache
Principal Acupoints: Zusanli (ST 36), Zhongwan (RN 12) and Neiguan (PC 6);
Supplemental Acupoints: Youmen (KI 21) and Zhangmen (LR 13)
Hyperhydrochloria
Principal Acupoints: Weishu (BL 21), Dachangshu (BL 25) and Neiguan (PC 6);
Supplemental Acupoints: Zusanli (ST 36) and Dazhu (BL 11)
Achlorhydria

Principal Acupoints: Ganshu (BL 18), Weishu (BL 21) and Zhongwan (RN 12);
Supplemental Acupoints: Neiguan (PC 6) and Zusanli (ST 36)

Diarrhea
Principal Acupoints: Tianshu (ST 25), Neiguan (PC 6) and Zusanli (ST 36);
Supplemental Acupoints: Qihai (RN 6) and Sanyinjiao (SP 6)

Constipation
Principal Acupoints: Zusanli (ST 36), Tianshu (ST 25) and Dachangshu (BL 25);
Supplemental Acupoints: Yanglingquan (GB 34) and Taibai (SP 3)

Incontinence of Stools
Principal Acupoints: Baliao (BL 30-33), Qihai (RN 6) and Guanyuan (RN 4);
Supplemental Acupoints: Zusanli (ST 36) and Mingmen (DU 4)

Hematemesis
Principal Acupoints: Daling (PC 7), Hegu (LI 4) and Qihai (RN 6);
Supplemental Acupoints: Zusanli (ST 36) and Neiguan (PC 6).

Ascitese
Principal Acupoints: Hegu (LI 4), Zusanli (ST 36) and Zhigou (SJ 6);
Supplemental Acupoints: Sanyinjiao (SP 6) and Neiguan (PC 6)

Diseases of Locomotive System

Pain and Impairment of Motor Function of Neck, Shoulder, Back, Lumbar and
Sacral Regions:

Nape of the Neck:
Principal Acupoints: Wangu (GB 12), Fengchi (GB 20) and Hegu (LI 4);
Supplemental Acupoints: Lieque (LU 7) and Dazhu (BL 11)

Suprascapular Region
Principal Acupoints: Dazhu (BL 11) and Jianjing (GB 21);
Supplemental Acupoints: Zhigou (SJ 6) and Waiguan (SJ 5)

Infrascapular Region
Principal Acupoints: Jianyu (LI 15) and Jianzhen (SI 9);
Supplemental Acupoints: Tianzong (SI 11) and Waiguan (SJ 5)

Back
Principal Acupoints: Chize (LU 5) and Weizhong (BL 40);
Supplemental Acupoints: Quchi (LI 11) and Luozhen (EX-point)

Lumbago
Principal Acupoints: Huantiao (GB 30) and Weizhong (BL 40);
Supplemental Acupoints: Renzhong (DU 26) and Yanglingquan (GB 34)

Sacrum
Principal Acupoints: Sanyinjiao (SP 6), Chengshan (BL 57) and Kunlun (BL 60);
Supplemental Acupoints: Huantiao (GB 30) and Weizhong (BL 40)

Upper Limb Pain

Forearm
Principal Acupoints: Neiguan (PC 6), Waiguan (SJ 5) and Quchi (LI 11);

Supplemental Acupoints: Hegu (LI 4) and Chize (LU 5)

Upper Arms

Principal Acupoints: Quchi (LI 11), Jianjing (GB 21) and Jianyu (LI 15);

Supplemental Acupoints: Hegu (LI 4) and Waiguan (SJ 5).

Lower Limb Pain

Legs

Principal Acupoints: Yangchi (SJ 4), Sanyinjiao (SP 6) and Yanglingquan (GB 34);

Supplemental Acupoints: Yinlingquan (SP 9) and Zusanli (ST 36)

Thighs

Principal Acupoints: Weizhong (BL 40), Fengshi (GB 31) and Huantiao (GB 30);

Supplemental Acupoints: Chengshan (BL 57) and Chengjing (BL 56)

Iliac Region

Principal Acupoints: Huantiao (GB 30), Biguan (ST 31) and Yanglingquan (GB 34);

Supplemental Acupoints: Weizhong (BL 40) and Fengshi (GB 31)

Ankle Joints

Principal Acupoints: Jinmen (BL 63), Kunlun (BL 60) and Zhaohai (KI 6);

Supplemental Acupoints: Chengjin (BL 56) and Pucan (BL 61)

Soles of the Feet

Principal Acupoints: Kunlun (BL 60), Yongquan (KI 1) and Zhaohai (KI 6);

Supplemental Acupoints: Jinmen (BL 63) and Pucan (BL 61)

Paralysis of Lower Limbs

The acupoints mentioned above in lower limb pain may be used alternately.

Diseases of Kidney and Urinary System

Frequent Micturition

Principal Acupoints: Zhongji (RN 3), Qihai (RN 6) and Guanyuan (RN 4);

Supplemental Acupoints: Sanyinjiao (SP 6) and Hegu (LI 4)

Anuria

Principal Acupoints: Qihai (RN 6), Zhongji (RN 3) and Guanyuan (RN 4);

Supplemental Acupoints: Shuidao (ST 28) and Mingmen (DU 4)

Renal Stone:

Principal Acupoints: Qihai (RN 6), Guanyuan (RN 4) and Zusanli (ST 36);

Supplemental Acupoints: Baliao (BL 30-33) and Mingmen (DU 4)

Emission

Principal Acupoints: Sanyinjiao (SP 6), Guanyuan (RN 4) and Zhongji (RN 3);

Supplemental Acupoints: Mingmen (DU 4) and Shenshu (BL 23)

Impotence:

Principal Acupoints: Sanyinjiao (SP 6), Guanyuan (RN 4) and Zhongji (RN 3);

Supplemental Acupoints: Mingmen (DU 4) and Shenshu (BL 23)

Diseases of Ear, Nose, Throat and Eyes

Tinnitus, Deafness and Ear Pain:
Principal Acupoints: Tinggong (SJ 10), Fengchi (GB 20) and Yifeng (SJ 17);
Supplemental Acupoints: Hegu (LI 4) and Zusanli (ST 36)

Nasal Bleeding
Principal Acupoints: Hegu (LI 4), Yingxiang (LI 20) and Dazhui (DU 14);
Supplemental Acupoints: Weizhong (BL 40) and Fengfu (DU 16)

Nasal Obstruction and Smelling Impairment
Principal Acupoints: Yingxiang (LI 20) and Shangxing (DU 23);
Supplemental Acupoints: Hegu (LI 4) and Renzhong (DU 26)

Conjunctiva Congestion:
Principal Acupoints: Jingming (BL 1), Sizhukong (SJ 23) and Tongziliao (GB 1);
Supplemental Acupoints: Hegu (LI 4) and Cuanzhu (BL 2)

Excessive Tears:
Principal Acupoints: Cuanzhu (BL 2), Fengchi (GB 20) and Hegu (LI 4);
Supplemental Acupoints: Taiyang (EX-HN 5) and Tongziliao (GB 1)

Syncope and Shock
Principal Acupoints: Shaoshang (LU 11), Renzhong (DU 26) and Shixuan
   (EX-UE 11);
Supplemental Acupoints: Neiguan (PC 6) and Yongquan (KI 1)

Convulsion:
Principal Acupoints: Hegu (LI 4), Shaoshang (LU 11) and Renzhong (DU 26);
Supplemental Acupoints: Shixuan (EX-UE 11) and Yongquan (KI 1)

Aphasia
Principal Acupoints: Yamen (DU 15), Dazhui (DU 14) and Zhigou (SJ 6);
Supplemental Acupoints: Yongquan (KI 1) and Zusanli (ST 36)

Gynaecological Diseases

Dysmenorrhea:
Principal Acupoints: Qihai (RN 6), Shangliao (BL 30) and Dachangshu (BL 25);
Supplemental Acupoints: Shenshu (BL 23) and Xuehai (SP 10)

Oligomenorrhea and Amenorrhea
Principal Acupoints: Sanyinjiao (SP 6), Hegu (LI 4) and Zhongji (RN 3);
Supplemental Acupoints: Xuehai (SP 10) and Mingmen (DU 4)

Profuse Menstration
Principal Acupoints: Qihai (RN 6), Guanyuan (RN 4) and Zusanli (ST 36);
Supplemental Acupoints: Yinbai (SP 1) and Weizhong (BL 40)

Profuse Leukorrhea
Principal Acupoints: Sanyinjiao (SP 6), Qihai (RN 6) and Shenshu (BL 23);
Supplemental Acupoints: Daimai (GB 26) and Zhongji (RN 3)

Chapter 6
CLINICAL PRACTICE OF QIGONG ACUPRESSURE THERAPY

Essentials of Qigong Acupressure Therapy

To produce a satisfactory therapeutic result, the techniques of qigong acupressure should be correctly selected in accordance with the nature of diseases, the condition of patients, the differential diagnosis of syndromes as well as the anatomical contours of the area of the body where acupressure will be applied. Before starting a qigong acupressure therapy session, the diagnosis of a disease should be correctly made by means of the four diagnostic methods and the eight diagnostic principles in order to understand whether the disease is superficial or deep, cold or hot and deficient or excessive in nature as well as which organs and meridians are involved. Without a correct diagnosis of the disease, the physician can not correctly select the adequate maneuvers and techniques (reinforcing or reducing) and accurately apply the appropriate stimulation (gentle or heavy) to effectively cure it.

The inspection, auscultation with olfaction, interrogation and palpation are the four main methods of diagnosis in traditional Chinese medicine; and the yin or yang, exterior or interior, deficient or excessive and cold or hot syndromes are the eight fundamental types of syndrome for differential diagnosis. The eight types of syndromes can be divided into two groups: The yin group contains the interior, deficient and cold syndromes; and the yang group contains the exterior, excessive and hot syndromes. The eight syndromes are closely linked with each other and they can simultaneously coexist, for example, some yin symptoms may appear in a yang syndrome and vice versa; external symptoms may be present in interior syndromes and vice versa; excessive and deficient symptoms may simultaneously coexist in a patient; and cold and hot symptoms may be mixed up.

According to the rules of differential diagnosis in traditional Chinese medicine, yang and hot syndromes usually show clinical manifestations of fever, evaporation, flaccidness, perspiration and annoyance; yin and cold syndromes manifest coldness, condensation, shrinkage, coagulation and blockage; deficient syndromes show manifest constriction, looseness, numbness and weakness; exterior syndromes usually show a nature of ascension; interior syndromes often show a nature of heaviness and descent. The transference of evils (pathogenic factors) along the meridians may cause a spread of disease from a superficial part to an interior part of the body; the movement of evils against the meridian flow indicates the evils are very violent; manifestations of sparseness and looseness indicate the deficiency in the patient; condensation indicates the accumulation of evils or stagnation of qi in the body; disordered clinical manifestations indicate a functional disturbance in the body; and the appearance of emotional disturbance, such as joy, angry, sadness, anxiety, grief and terror indicates the invasion of evils from internal organs into the brain.

In addition, the internal organs may affect the color of the body surface. For example, normal heart qi may displays a red color, lung qi shows a white color, spleen and stomach qi produces a yellowish-green color, liver qi displays a dark green color, gallbladder qi shows a blue color and kidney qi produces a purple color. The qi of internal organs is clear, clean and transparent in healthy subjects; but it is turbid, dark and grayish in unhealthy patients. From the change of color on the body surface, the injury of internal organs and the severity of diseases may be diagnosed and estimated.

Therapeutic Methods for Different Syndromes

Exterior Syndromes:
(1) Local Lesions: Rubbing and kneading with activated qi for soft tissue injury and vibrating with activated qi for muscle and bone injuries.
(2) General Symptoms: Finger-pressing and rubbing with activated qi for febrile diseases.
Interior Syndromes:
(1) Interior-excessive Syndromes: Reducing technique using finger- or palm-pressing, grasping, patting and pinching with activated qi.
(2) Interior-deficient Syndromes: Reinforcing technique using pressing, kneading, rubbing and pinching the muscles along the spine with activated qi.
Deficient Syndromes: Reinforcing technique using gentle maneuvers with activated qi for a long duration.
Excessive Syndromes: Reducing technique using quick, deep and forcible pressing, rubbing and finger-pressing with activated qi for a short duration.
Hot Syndromes: Qigong acupressure is applied on the meridians, in the opposite direction of natural qi flow.
Cold Syndromes: Qigong acupressure is rhythmically applied on the meridians, following direction of natural qi flow.

Qigong Acupressure Therapy on Different Parts of the Body

Qigong Acupressure Therapy on the Head

Qigong acupressure on the head is a common health maintenance therapy. According to traditional medical theory, "yang from all over the body assembles at the head." Diseases of head may be caused by various etiological factors; for example, headaches may be caused by wind and cold evils, blockage of clear yang, tiredness and consumption of qi, deficiency of yin and blood, deficiency of qi and blood, adverse ascension of liver yang with dizziness, cerebral contussion and sequelae of cerebral thrombosis.

(1) Daoyin qi (induce and motivate qi):

Patients lie on their back with the body relaxed and eyes closed. Put your hand over the head of the patient and to repeatedly flex and extend the joints to *daoyin* qi over Baihui (DU 20) to adjust yin and yang and to relieve meridian blockages in the patient's body.

(2) Rubbing Along Bilateral Superciliary Arches:

Patients lie on their back with the body relaxed and eyes closed. Use your thumb pads (with activated qi) to rub from the Yintang (EX-HN 3) point along the upper border of the superciliary arches to the bilateral Taiyang (EX-HN 5) points. The initial pressure should be sufficiently heavy and an even pressure is maintained through the rubbing session to produce a soft and comfortable sensation. The erasing may also be applied along three to five vertical parallel lines from the forehead to occiput [Fengchi (GB 20)] or along three horizontal lines over the forehead of the patient 6-12 times. This will open the "doors" and "skylight windows" of the skull and improve brain functioning and eyesight, tonify yang and tranquilize the mind.

(3) Pushing Around the Eyeballs:

Patients lie on their back with the body relaxed and eyes closed. Use your thumb pads to push (with activated qi) from Cuanzhu (BL 2) along the upper border of the superciliary arches through Yuyao (EX-HN 4) to Taiyang (EX-HN 5) 6-12 times to improve eyesight.

(4) Pressing Around the Eyeballs:

Patients lie on their back with the body relaxed and eyes closed. Use the thumb pads (with activated qi) to press Jingming (UB 1), outer canthus, Ermen (SJ 21), Tinggong (SI 19) and Tinghui (GB 2) points 6-12 times; and then along the lower border of the occipital bone press bilateral Fengchi (GB 20) to produce a sore, hot and distending sensation which may be radiated forward from this point. This treatment may improve vision and hearing and relieve headaches.

(5) Comb Hair and Scratch Scalp:

Patients lie on their back with the body relaxed and eyes closed. Your fingers are flexed and the finger pads are used (with activated qi) to quickly comb and scratch the scalp with enough pressure 6-12 times to eliminate evils wind, tonify the brain, refresh the mind and improve mental functions.

Qigong Acupressure Therapy on the Neck

In clinical practice symptoms of the neck are commonly present in many diseases, such as cervical spondylopathy, stiff neck, cervicoscapular syndrome, etc. The nape of the neck and Yuzhen (BL 9) is an important region in qigong exercise and acupressure therapy, because there are many meridians passing and crisscrossing this region, constantly moving qi which can be utilized for exercise and treatment of diseases. Qigong acupressure therapy on the neck encompasses the following methods:

Techniques

(1) Pressing Fengchi (GB 20): Patients lie on their stomach and you use the finger pads (with activated qi) to press and knead Fengchi (GB 20) to eliminate wind and cold evils and to cure headaches and common colds.

(2) Grasping Yuzhen (BL 9): Place your palm (with activated qi) over Yuzhen (BL 9) and grasp the nape muscles with the five fingers and then pluck the muscles with the thumb to remove blood stasis in meridians and stop pain.

Qigong Acupressure Therapy on the Chest and Abdomen

The therapeutic results of qigong acupressure therapy for chest and abdominal diseases are impressive: it can improve the functioning of the spleen and stomach, and adjust circulation of qi and expand chest cavity to cure stomachaches, lower abdominal pain, chest and intercostal pain, dysmenorrhea, constipation, diarrhea, ptosis of internal organs and postoperative adhesions.

Techniques

(1) Pushing the Chest: Patients lie on their back with the knee joints flexed or extended. Stand at the patient's head. A force is transferred distally from your palm and applied by two extended fingers (with activated qi) to Tiantu (RN 22); and then the fingers are used to gently push along the Ren Meridian to Danzhong (RN 17). Again, from the center of the sternum the pressing is continuously applied along a horizontal direction to bilateral Yunmen (LU 2) to expand the chest cavity, adjust circulation of qi, relieve chest distress, and adjust the disturbance of respiration.

(2) Regulating Intercostal Spaces: Patients lie on their back with the knee joints flexed or extended. Stand at the patient's head. Your fingers are separated from each other and firmly put into the intercostal spaces to apply pressure (with activated qi) into the chest, and then the fingers are pushed laterally to the subaxillary region. The regulating methods should be applied from the upper chest downward to relax the intercostal muscles, adjust the functioning of the liver and gallbladder and to treat asthma.

(3) Kneading and Vibrating Abdomen: Patients lie on their back with the knee joints flexed or extended. Stand at the patient's head. The proximal part (thenar and hypothenar prominence) of your palm is used to apply vibrating pressure and at the same time slowly knead the abdomen in a clockwise direction 6-12 times. This treats constipation, diarrhea, intestinal adhesion and ptosis of the stomach with satisfactory results. The pressure should be applied steadily and gently.

(4) Palm-kneading Around Umbilicus: Patients lie on their back with the knee joints flexed or extended. Stand at the patient's head. Your palm is used to knead the abdomen in a clockwise direction around the umbilicus and then to knead the abdomen in a counterclockwise direction 12-24 times, or until the patient feels hot in his or her abdomen. The method may be used to treat stomach ache and abdominal pain and swelling, and it is also useful to relieve postoperative abdominal swelling.

Qigong Acupressure Therapy on the Back and Lumbar Regions

Lumbago is a common disease caused by many pathogenic factors. Traditional Chinese physicians believe there is a close relation between lumbago and the kidney. As mentioned in ancient medical books that the waist is an important articulation of the trunk and the body can not freely turn and bend, if the waist is injured. According to the ancient medical book *General Treatise on Causes and Symptoms of Diseases*, lumbago is caused by wind and dampness evils, deficiency of the kidney and external trauma.

Techniques

Patients lie on the abdomen with cushions put underneath the chest, abdomen and knees to relax the back muscles. The qigong practioner stands beside the patient.

(1) Kneading the Back: Use your palm (with activated qi concentrated at the inner Luogong (PC 8)) to knead the back from Dazhui (DU 14) downward to Yaoyangguan (DU 3), and again from Dazhu (BL 11) downward along bilateral Urinary Bladder Meridians 6-12 times. This will remove stasis in the meridians, connect the exterior and interior organs of the body and relieve pain.

(2) Pressing Acupoints and Tender Spots on the Back: Use your thumb pads to apply pressure to the bilateral Fengmen (BL 12) points of the Urinary Bladder Meridian, and then move downward applying pressure to tender spots on the way to Baliao (BL 30-33). Do this 6-12 times to produce the same effects as mentioned above. The pressure applied to the acupoints and tender spots should be light and gentle to produce a tingling, numb, hot and distending sensation.

(3) Patting the Back: Use a palm to repeatedly pat the spinal column of the patient from the upper part of the back downward for 4-8 minutes. This produces a warm sensation. The patting may be also applied with both palms (alternately) to the tender spots in the lumbar and hip regions, as well as to the muscles of lower limbs. This strengthens the muscles and bones, removes stasis in the meridians, promotes circulation of qi and blood and tonifies internal organs.

(4) Bone Manipulation:

a. Over-extend Waist by Pulling Knee Joint Backward: Patients lie on their abdomen. Qigong practioner uses one hand to press the waist downward and use the other hand to support the opposite knee joint and forcibly pull it upward and backward to overextend and twist the waist until a cracking sound is produced. Repeat on the other leg. Then the palm-pressing technique is applied to Huantiao (GB 30) and the grasping is applied to Chengshan (BL 57), Kunlun (BL 60) and Jinmen (BL 63). This method is used to treat the acute muscular sprain of lower back and the subluxation of small vertebral joints.

b. Extending and Flexing Hip and Knee Joints: Patients lie on their backs with the muscles of their whole body relaxed and the qigong practioner uses one hand to hold the ankle joint of the patient and the other to support the same leg; then flex the hip and knee joints and rotate the hip joint back and forth 3-4 times; finally stretch and slowly pull the leg downward. The same procedure may be repeated on both legs, alternately, 3-4 times. Then press and knead the muscles of the thigh and leg to release the spasm. All the methods used in this treatment should be performed gently and steadily.

Notes and Suggestions

After spasms of the back and lumbar muscles are relieved by the above proce-dures, finger-pressing and kneading with activated qi may be repeatedly applied to the tender spots and nodules to produce a hot sensation in the patient. The above-mentioned manipulations are usually adopted to treat common lumbago, but for the lumbago due to some specific diseases the treatment procedure should be modified: for example, pressing and kneading with activated qi are the best choice for patients with muscular rheumatism of the back, but the overextending for the waist should not be used on them; the push-rubbing and patting are a better choice for patients with hypertrophic spondilitis; the overextending for the waist may be applied to patients with muscular strain of the lower back; and the overextending for the waist should be used as the chief treatment in patients with subluxation of small lumbar vertebral joints. Patients should take a sitting posture during this treatment. The cracking sound produced by this procedure indicates a good therapeutic result has been obtained.

Qigong Acupressure Therapy on the Four Limb Joints

Techniques

Patients take a supine posture with knee joint extended or take a sitting posture with the knee joint flexed and the qigong practioner stands beside the patient to treat them with finger-pressing, vibrating, palm-pressing, pushing, grasping, rotating, shaking or streching.

Notes and Suggestions

The qigong acupressure methods for the four limb joints are about the same, although the joints have different locations, size, functions and activities. Qigong acupressure is an effective therapy for sprains, contusions, lacerations and rheuma-tism of joints, because it can promote circulation of qi and blood, remove stasis in the meridians, correct displacement of tendons and bones and faciliate movement of the joints. Traditional Chinese physicians believe that acupressure applied along the meridians can relieve qi blockages; and that massage applied to lesions with stasis and coagulation of blood may resolve the local swelling caused by stagnation and accumulation. Acupoints arround the joints are used in acupressure therapy to treat diseases of those joints: for example, Xuehai (SP 10), Liangqiu (ST 34), lateral and medial Xiyan (ST 35 and EX-LE 4), Yinlingquan (SP 9), Yanglingquan (GB 34) and Weizhong (BL 40) points are commonly used to treat diseases of the knee joints.

Qigong Acupressure Therapy for Common Diseases

Qigong acupressure can be used to treat many medical, surgical, gynaecological, pediatric and traumatic diseases.

Headaches

Causes and Symptoms

The headache is a common subjective symptom and it often appears in many diseases caused by invasion of external evils, emotional strains, deficiency of qi and stasis of blood. Because the yang qi all over the body, the essence and blood in the five internal organs of the body are all transported to the head to nourish the brain, the acupoints on the head are particularly sensitive to qigong acupressure stimulation and it may produce a satisfactory therapeutic results for headaches.

Diagnosis and Treatment

(1) Headache Due to Common Colds:

Symptoms: Patients may suffer from a severe headache, chills, fever, cough, runny nose and soreness and weakness in the joints.

Therapeutic Techniques: Use finger pressing, palm pressing or grasping along both sides of spinal column, and palm pressing, kneading or grasping to muscles of the shoulder and arm. Repeat 3-5 times.

Healing Effects: The treatment can release stasis in the meridians, adjust qi and blood, relieve blood stasis, expel cold evil wind and stop pain.

(2) Headaches Due to Attacks of Evil Wind in the Meridians:

Symptoms: Patients may suffer from a pricking pain in the head with local swelling is commonly known as a migraine headache.

Therapeutic Techniques: According to the location of the headache, acupressure should be applied along the Yangming Meridian for frontal headaches and pain over superciliary arch; along the Jueyin Meridian for parietal headaches; along the Taiyang Meridian for occipital headaches; and along the Shaoyang Meridian for temporal headaches.

Healing Effects: The treatment can disperse evil wind, stop pain and remove stasis in the meridians.

Treatment Procedure

Patients lie on their back with eyes closed; the qigong practioner stands at the patient's head and applys the finger-pressing with activated qi to the acupoints of the head (selected according to the nature and location of the disease) and then to grasps the muscles along the shoulder and arm 6-12 times.

Notes and Suggestions

The headaches in patients with the common cold can be quickly relieved by qigong acupressure therapy. If the headache can not be alleviated or relieved by qigong acupressure, the patient should be carefully examined to find out the cause of the headaches which would require other treatment.

Case Report

Mr. Wang, a 24-year old student, first visited a clinic on June 8 1986. For one year the patient had suffered migraine or neurogenic headaches and excessively dreamful sleep. The headache was distending in nature and aggravated by reading and studying in the recent half year. Sleep was also interrupted by the headache attacks. A neurological examination did not show any abnormality. After qigong acupressure therapy was applied 6 times, the headache and other sufferings were almost completely relieved.

Vertigo

Causes and Symptoms

Vertigo is a common subjective symptom caused by many pathogenic factors and it is known as periperal vertigo in modern medicine. In patients with mild vertigo, sufferings may be relieved after a short rest in bed with eyes closed. Severe cases may suffer from a serious rotatory vertigo, like sea and air sickness and they can not stand stable and straight. As mentioned by ancient physicians, vertigo is usually caused by yin deficiency and stirring up of internal liver wind or by head trauma. In excessive cases, vertigo is caused by phlegm-fire or wind-phlegm. The symptoms of vertigo can be alleviated or relieved by qigong acupressure therapy.

Diagnosis and Treatment

(1) Deficiency of Qi and Blood:

Symptoms: Patients may suffer from rotatory vertigo, blurred vision or dark blindness, tinnitus and weakness of the whole body.

Therapeutic Techniques: The kneading method with activated qi along the Ren and Du meridians and the pressing with activated qi at the middle and lower Dantian.

Healing Effects: The treatment can enrich qi and blood and promote blood circulation for relieving vertigo.

(2) Adverse Ascension of Liver Yang:

Symptoms: Patients may suffer from severe dizziness with a splitting sensation in the head, and soreness and weakness of the waist and legs caused by emotional upset and anger.

Therapeutic Techniques: Acupressure with activated qi is applied along the Du Meridian through the upper Dantian, parietal and occipital parts of the head.

Healing Effects: The treatment can disperse and discharge adversely ascending yang and tonify the liver and kidney.

(3) Internal Blockage by Phlegm and Dampness:

Symptoms: Patients may suffer from chest pain and distress, nausea, vomiting, poor appetite and tiredness of the body.

Therapeutic Techniques: Routine qigong acupressure therapy over the chest and abdomen and the kneading method with activated qi along Meridians of Foot-Yangming.

Healing Effects: The treatment can warm yang qi, resolve dampness, raise clear qi up and bring turbid qi down.

Techniques

Besides the therapeutic methods mentioned in the paragraph of differential diagnosis and treatment, the pressing, finger-kneading, push-rubbing and grasping methods may also be used to treat this disease.

Treatment Procedure

Patients take a sitting (or supine) posture. Stand behind the patient and use thumb-kneading with activated qi along the Du Meridian from the head to the lower back 3-6 times. After the muscles are relaxed and the patient feels comfortable, other methods may be applied according to the practical condition. Pressure should be applied evenly and flexibly by appropriately combining pressing and kneading methods. The reinforcing or reducing technique should be correctly selected and pressure applied on the patient should be not very violent. The treatment may be applied once or twice a day. One therapeutic course contains 12 treatments and the second course may be started after a week of rest.

Notes and Suggestions

Qigong acupressure should be performed from the upper body downward and from the medial part to the lateral part of the body. Pressing and kneading along the meridians can push qi and blood flow downward to refresh the mind and improve eyesight; and the grasping can relieve stasis of qi and blood in blood vessels and promote their circulation, thus reducing and relieving vertigo.

Case Report

Ms. Su, an officer in Overseas Chinese Office of Fujian Province, first visited a clinic in June 1982. For five years the patient had suffered from dizziness, tinnitus, blurred vision, insomnia and excessively dreamful sleep. The disease was first caused by overfatigue and nervous tension and drugs could not cure it. On the first visit a diagnosis of peripheral vertigo was made. After qigong acupressure with external qi was applied 6 times, the symptoms were much improved; they were almost entirely relieved after another 6 treatments. Self-treatment of qigong acupressure was taught to the patient and she was asked to continue the treatment on her own to maintain her positive therapeutic results.

Fainting

Causes and Symptoms

Fainting is a common syndrome with a clinical manifestation of sudden falling down, temporary loss of consciousness, disturbance of locomotive functions and coma. It does not have the common sequelae of cerebral accident, such as hemiplegia, aphasia or deviation of eyes and mouth angle after the recovery of consciousness. Qigong acupressure therapy is very useful to promote the recovery of consciousness and to rescue the life of comatose patients.

Diagnosis and Treatment

Fainting can be divided into three types:

(1) Common Fainting:

Symptoms: Some prodromal symptoms may appear before the loss of consciousness, including dizziness, blurred vision, palpitation of the heart, vomiting and cold sweating. The pulse is weak.

Therapeutic Techniques: The grasping technique with activated qi to the muscle beside Daying (ST 5) (sterno-cleidomastoid muscle) and the back muscles and the finger-pressing technique to Renzhong (DU 26) and other acupoints.

Healing Effects: The treatment can refresh mind, open orifices and cure collapse.

(2) Fainting Due to Heat Stroke:

Symptoms: Patients may suffer from the symptoms of heat stroke, including profuse sweating, thrist and weakness of limbs.

Therapeutic Techniques: Use the grasping technique to the muscle beside Daying (ST 5) (sterno-cleidomastoid muscle) and the posterior group of muscles (extersors) of the arm to promote circulation of qi through meridians.

Healing Effects: The treatment can eliminate heat stroke, tonify qi, clear heat and refresh the mind.

(3) Coma Due to Blockage of Phlegm:

Symptoms: Patients may suffer from critical symptoms, including obstruction of throat by accumulated phlegm, and chest distress and distention.

Therapeutic Techniques: Use the grasping with activated qi to the medial group of muscles of the thighs and the posterior-medial group of muscles (calf muscles) of the legs.

Healing Effects: The treatment can soothe the liver, stop blowing of liver wind, transfer phlegm downward and open orifices.

Techniques

Besides the techniques mentioned above, the finger-pressing, pinching, palm-pressing and kneading with activated qi may also be applied to treat the patients.

Treatment Procedure

Patients take a supine posture with the coat unbuttoned; the head is cushioned on a pillow or resting flat. When the activated qi is moved to the fingers pinch Shuigou (DU 26), Hegu (LI 4) and the tip of patient's middle finger and then press and knead the patient's superciliary arches.

Notes and Suggestions

After the conciousness is restored by qigong acupressure therapy, routine qigong acupressure over the chest and abdomen may be applied to adjust the functions of Sanjiao (Three Energizers), tonify the qi of Zhongjiao (Middle Energizer), strengthen body resistance and to enrich vital energy. In addition, for obtaining a better therapeutic result, the fainting patient should be moved to an environment with good ventilation for better treatment and recovery.

The grasping pressure should be firm and gentle. It is combined with a plucking action and the activated qi to produce better results. The grasping and plucking can not be applied to the big blood and lymph vessels. In patients with incontinence of urine and deep coma not controllable by qigong acupressure therapy, other specific emergent treatments must be adopted to save the patient's life.

Case Report

Mr. Li, a 48-year-old peasant from Hebei Province, first visited a clinic in July 1978. Because of exhausting farm work, the patient suddenly fell down and lost consciousness. Upon physical examination, he was in a comatose condition and could not move; but after one emergent qigong acupressure treatment, his consciousness was soon restored. After a course of treatment once a day for 6 days, the patient completely recovered.

Asthma

Causes and Symptoms

Asthma is usually an excessive disease caused by wind, cold, heat or phlegm evils.

(1) Patients suffering from the excessive type often have shortness of breath and chest distress with thick, sticky phlegm. This condition is usually aggravated in cold seasons.

(2) Patients suffering from the deficient type may have shortness of breath and palpitation of the heart with thin, sticky, foamy phlegm. This condition is usually aggravated by physical exertion.

Techniques

Routine qigong acupressure therapy on the neck, chest and abdomen is usually applied with pressing, pushing, grasping and finger-pressing techniques.

Treatment Procedure

(1) Patients take a sitting posture and the qigong practioner stands beside them and uses the radial border of thumb with activated qi to push along an oblique line from the lower pole of the ear root to Quepen (ST 12) on both sides 6-12 times; and then rub the forehead and grasp the nape of the diseased side [around Fengchi (GB 20) and Fengfu (DU 16)] 3-6 times.

(2) Stand beside the patient and use a relaxing technique to push and press the upper chest, spleen and stomach as well as the back and loins; and then apply the finger-pressing technique at the Feishu (BL 13), Shenshu (BL 23) and Mingmen (DU 4) points to produce a hot and relaxing sensation.

(3) Patients take a sitting posture or lie on their stomach. Stand beside them and apply pushing and grasping with activated qi along the spinal column from Dazhui (DU 14) to Fengfu (DU 16) to produce a hot and relaxing sensation.

Notes and Suggestions

(1) The therapeutic effect of qigong acupressure is better in patients who have had this disease for a short time and their health is easier to restore; but in chronic patients the improvement of the disease treated by qigong acupressure is usually incomplete and takes time.

(2) Patients should do physical exercise to strengthen their physique and enhance their body resistance, but the exercise must not be very strenuous.

(3) Cold, raw, greasy or spicy food, as well as smoking and alcohol, should be avoided and patients should pay extra attention to keeping their body warm and protecting themselves from common cold attacks caused by a sudden change of weather.

Case Reports

(1) Mr. Wei, 66 years old and the president of an art college, first visited a clinic in November 1982. For six years the patient experienced repeated attacks of asthma and dyspnea. In recent years, the patient suffered from shortness of breath, puffing and cough with sticky phlegm. Severe attacks of asthma could not controlled by drugs, but after qigong acupressure therapy applied 12 times, the above symptoms were almost entirely relieved. To maintaining this good therapeutic result the patient was asked to consistantly perform the *tuna* (respiratory) and physical exercise. The patient had no more asthmatic attacks.

(2) Dr. Pan, a 35-year-old woman physician, first visited a clinic in October 1990. For ten years the patient had had endured repeated attacks of asthma and orthopnea. The patient suffered from dyspnea, which was especially bad at night; she could not lie flat to sleep. Attacks were also serious in cold season and after physical exertion. The patient had a family histroy of asthma. Asthma attacks could not be controlled by drugs, but after qigong acupressure therapy was applied 12 times, all her sufferings were abolished and she had no asthma attacks.

Insomnia

Causes and Symptoms

Patients with insomnia can not quickly fall asleep or maintain a stable and sound sleep at night. The manifestations of insomnia are varied: in some patients sleep may be very shallow, excessively dreamful, easily interrupted. It may also be difficult to fall asleep. Some patients may be repeatedly awakened but capable of falling asleep again for many times throughout the night. In addition, patients with insomnia may also suffer from poor memory and fits of terror.

Diagnosis and Treatment

(1) Deficiency of Heart and Spleen:

Symptoms: Deficiency of the heart and spleen due to severe worry may cause shallow and excessively dreamful sleep, palpitation of the heart, poor memory and frequent spontaneous sweating.

Therapeutic Techniques: Pressing and kneading with activated qi applied to the back acupoints: such as Xinshu (BL 15), Pishu (BK 20), Weishu (BL 21) and Jueyinshu (BL 14) points or along the Foot-Jueyin and Foot-Yangming meridians.

Healing Effects: The treatment can tonify heart, strengthen spleen and stomach and tranquilize the mind.

(2) Dissociation of Heart and Kidney:

Symptoms: Weakness of the kidneys due to very frequent sexual activities may cause dizziness, tinnitus, emission and soreness of back.

Therapeutic Techniques: Pressing with activated qi applied along the Hand- and Foot-Shaoyin Meridians 6-12 times.

Healing Effects: The treatment can tonify heart, strengthen the kidneys and maintain balance between fire and water (heart and kidney).

(3) Upward Stirring of Liver Yang:

Symptoms: The functional disturbance of the spleen due to mental depression may cause pain and distention of the chest, mental hyperirritability, fury, dizziness and headaches.

Healing Effects: The treatment can reduce excessiveness of the liver, strengthen the spleen and stomach and tranquilize the mind.

Techniques

Besides the therapeutic methods mentioned in the paragraph of diagnosis and treatment, routine qigong acupressure therapy in the head region is often used to treat insomnia.

Treatment Procedure

(1) Patients take a supine posture. Apply routine qigong acupressure therapy on the head 6-12 times; and then the pressing is applied along several meridians, especially the Shaoyang Meridians from the upper body downward. A therapeutic course is once a day for 6-12 days; the second course may be started after a rest of 7-15 days.

(2) Patients lie on their stomach. Apply massage and rubbing with activated qi using the palm over the spinal column and pinching the mudcles along the spine 3-5 times; and then the finger-pressing is applied to the meridians several times.

Notes and Suggestions

To obtain a good effect, it is best to apply qigong acupressure 1-2 hours before the patient goes to bed; continue treatment until the patient falls asleep. For chronic patients, the causes of insomnia should be removed and qigong and physical exercise should be regularly performed to maintain positive therapeutic results.

Case Report

Mrs. Li, a 61-year-old officer, first visited a clinic in June 1985. For ten years the patient suffered from insomnia and excessively dreamful and easily interrupted sleep. She slept only 2-3 hours a night. After 6 treatments of qigong acupressure therapy with application of external qi, she could sleep 4-6 hours per night, and, after 12 treatments, the insomnia was almost cured. Two years after the initial treatment we contacted the patient and learned that her positive therapeutic result had been maintained.

Vomiting

Causes and Symptoms

If there are no organic pathological changes in the patient, vomiting, as a disease similar to neurogenic vomiting or gastro-intestinal neurosis in modern medicine is caused by emotional disturbance, but traditional Chinese medicine sees the cause as an invasion of liver qi into the spleen. The main symptoms are repeated bouts of regular or periodical vomiting with mucous and bile vomitus. The vomiting is not very troublesome and the vomit is not very difficult to throw up. Severe cases may also suffer from headaches, dizziness, lassitude and poor appetite.

Techniques

Finger-pressing, pinching, pushing, kneading and knocking techniques with activated qi are used.

Treatment Procedure

(1) Acupressure (finger-pressing): Patients take a supine posture and the qigong practioner stands beside them to do acupressure (finger-pressing) with activated qi to Jinghou (EX-point), on Fengchi (GB 20) and Rutu (EX-point) as the principal points; and then to bilateral Neiguan (PC 6) as a supplemental point to produce a hot and comfortable sensation in the stomach.

(2) Push-kneading: First pinch the base of the finger nails and toe nails and Achilles tendon of the patient and then use the thumb or the proximal part of the palm to push and knead spaces between the 9th and 10th ribs (on the subaxillary lines).

(3) Knocking: First move qi to the tips of the fingers and use them to knock Jiuwei (RN 15) and Juque (RN 14) and then to push-knead them. The finger-pressing is applied to bilateral Zusanli (ST 36) as a supplemental point to adjust the functions of spleen and stomach.

Notes and Suggestions

(1) Physical Exercise: Patients should regularly perform physical exercise to strengthen their physique and maintain health.

(2) Diet and Sleep Control: Patients should adjust and improve their dietary and sleeping habits and eliminate harmful factors which affect their mental and emotional mood.

Case Report

Mr. Jiao, a 51-year-old patient from Hebei Province, first visited a clinic in August 1976. He complained of vomiting, lassitude, headaches, dizziness and poor appetite, but the clinical and laboratory examinations did not show any evidences of organic pathological changes. After qigong acupressure therapy and three applications of external qi, vomiting, headaches and dizziness were much improved and they were almost completely relieved after 6 subsequent treatments.

Hiccups

Causes and Symptoms

Hiccups are usually caused by accumulation and blockage of pathogenic factors and disturbed circulation of vital energy after violent rage or improper use of drugs. At such times, the stomach qi and diaphragm can not be normally spread out and moved downward, causing short, repeated hiccups.

Techniques

Palm-pressing, rubbing, finger-pressing and grasping techniques with activated qi are used along the Hand-Jueyin Meridian and pinching at Hegu (LI 4) or finger-pressing at Quepen (ST 12).

Treatment Procedure

(1) Patients take a supine posture and the qigong practioner stands beside them

and presses and rubs with activated qi from the sternum, Huagai (RN 20) and Danzhong (RN 17) points downward to induce and motivate qi to the lower Dantian; then rub downward along the ribs 6-12 times; and finally press and knead along the Ren Meridian to umbilicus and motivate qi to the bilateral Yongquan (KI 1) point.

(2) Patients take a sitting posture and the physician stands behind grasping the scapular muscles with activated qi and pressing Tianzong (SI 11) with the finger. At the same time, the patient is asked to hold their breath for 1-3 minutes. Then grasp the Hand-Jueyin Meridians and press the Dazhu (BL 11), Feishu (BL 13), Xinshu (BL 15) and Geshu (BL 17) points successively with the finger.

Notes and Suggestions

(1) Qigong acupressure can effectively stop hiccups because it can disperse out and move down stagnated and disturbed qi, expand the chest cavity, adjust circulation of qi and release diaphragm spasms.

(2) The usage proven herbs formulas can also control hiccups. Occasional hiccups due to attacks of cold weather or before bowel movement in babies may be relieved by drinking hot water or performing qigong exercises.

Case Report

Mr. Su, a 62-year-old cadre, was admitted to a hospital in October 1984 for treatment of many diseases. During a long hospitalization and after the administration of many drugs, he developed hiccups with dyspnea and distress of the chest. After six qigong acupressure treatments (6 minutes for each treatment), the hiccups and other symptoms were alleviated; and after 12 treatments, the symptoms almost entirely disappered.

Toothaches

Causes and Symptoms

Toothaches may be due to excessive fire, deficient fire or wind fire. Patients with heat in the Yangming Meridian may experience thirst (with a desire to drink cold water) and constipation; patients with a deficiency of kidney water and a flaming-up of deficient fire may suffer toothaches of all teeth; and in patients with a chronic deficiency of yin and internal fire derived from wind evil toothaches may spread to the face.

Techniques

Finger-pressing, palm-pressing, rubbing and kneading techniques with activated qi.

Treatment Procedure

(1) Patients take a sitting or supine posture and the qigong practioner stands beside the patient and rubs their face on the diseased side (with activated qi) to relax the muscles. For toothaches of the upper jaw, finger-pressing is first applied to the acupoints of hand Taiyang and Shaoyang meridians on the face, such as Xiaguan (ST 7) point with the activated qi; and for toothache of lower jaw the acupoints on the hand Yangming meridian over lower jaw are pressed with finger for 6-12 times to

clear heat, expel wind, protect teeth and stop pain.

(2) For toothaches on one side, Hegu (LI 4) on the opposite side is pressed with the finger using activated qi for 3-5 minutes at the same time the patient is asked to make deep respirations.

Notes and Suggestions

In traditional Chinese medicine common causes of toothaches are wind-fire and decayed tooth. The neurogenic toothache in modern dental medicine is the same as the wind-fire toothache in traditional medicine. As proved by the clinical practice, qigong acupressure can definitely control toothaches, but it is only a temporary cure in patients with toothaches due to decayed tooth.

Case Report

A 14-year-old sportsman first visited a clinic in May 1985 because of a bad toothache caused by an attack of wind and cold evils after exhausting physical training. Intake of food and sleep were severely interfered with. A physical examination revealed sensitive left-side teeth and red, swollen gums. After the patient sat down and relaxed, qigong acupressure was applied; his toothache soon stopped. The swelling and gum pain was also relieved after a treatment applied on the second day.

Myopia

Causes and Symptoms

Short-sighted vision is a common eye disease, especially in youths. It is usually caused by bad reading habits or inappropriate illumination (too bright or too dark) or related hereditary defects. In traditional Chinese medicine this condition is believed to be related to liver and kidney organs and caused by tiredness from using eyes.

Techniques

Finger-pressing, bilateral rubbing, finger-vibrating and push-kneading techniques with activated qi.

Treatment Procedure

(1) Patients take a sitting or supine posture and the qigong practioner stands beside, evenly pushing (using activated qi) the Du, Taiyang and Shaoyang meridians on the head with the thumb 6-12 times.

(2) To rub (with activated qi) along the bilateral superciliary arches to Taiyang (EX-HN 5) 6-12 times; and then push and knead the Taiyang points.

(3) Patients take a supine or sitting posture with eyes closed and the qigong practioner stands at the head of the patient and presses the acupoints around the eyes with the middle finger using activated qi to produce a hot and bright sensation in the eyes; and then finger-pressing is at the applied bilateral Hegu (LI 4) points for 3-5 minutes to tonify the kidney and liver, promote blood circulation and improve eyesight.

Notes and Suggestions

(1) When applying acupressure around the eyes, the eye balls must be carefully

protected from accidental injury.

(2) False (acquired) myopia can be successfully cured by qigong acupressure therapy, but in chronic patients with myopia due to hereditary defects, qigong acupressure can only relieve some symptoms and control the progression of near-sightedness.

(3) After qigong acupressure therapy, patients should rest with their eyes closed and must not use their eyes to read books or watch television for a while.

(4) Patients should adopt a correct posture when reading books, and use good illumination. It is also important to rest the eyes after reading or watching for a long time and to perform the healing exercises for eyes (see Chapter 3).

Case Report

Miss Li, a 15-year-old student, visited a clinic with a chief complaint of blurred vision and reduced visual acuity over the last one and a half years. Her parents had a good eyesight. Besides nearsightedness, the patient also suffered from tiredness and distension of the eyes. Ophthalmological examinations showed a visual acuity of 0.3, and the outer eye structures were all normal. A diagnosis of myopia of both eyes was made. After 18 qigong acupressure treatments with activated qi, she was able to see comparatively clearer and her visual acuity was improved to 0.8. The distension and tiredness of eyes was also relieved.

Stiff Necks

Causes and Symptoms

Stiff necks are due to poor sleeping posture or by the blockage of qi and blood caused by attacks of wind and cold evils at the neck and back muscls. The main symptoms of this disease unilateral pain and stiffness of the neck muscles (bilateral involvement is very rare), deviation of the head to one side and limited neck movement. Patients with severe stiff neck may have severe pain radiating to the shoulder and back.

Techniques

Routine qigong acupressure therapy on the neck and the finger-pressing, palm-pressing, rubbing, pinching, grasping and plucking techniques with activated qi.

Treatment Procedure

(1) Grasping and Pinching Techniques: Patients take a sitting posture. Stand behind the patient and pinch the *jingban jin* (trapezius and supraspinous muscles) with the thumb and index fingers (with activated qi) and rub the diseased side of the neck with the proximal part of the palm 6-12 times. This helps release muscles spasms.

(2) Pressing and Rubbing Techniques: Use the right hand to press and rub the Du Meridian from the hair line over the nape region to the upper back. Use the thumb to press and knead stiff muscles on the diseased side with vibrations and activated qi 6-12 times. This helps release muscular spasms, promote blood circulation, remove blood stasis and stop pain. The pressure applied to the diseased part

should be adequate in strength.

(3) Skillful Twisting Technique: Ask the patient to relax their muscles and move the chin slightly downward. Use one hand to support the chin and another hand to hold the cheek. Without forewarning, quickly twist the neck within a limited range to the diseased side. This will produce a clicking (or cracking) sound from the joints. Patients may feel a sudden release of restriction and the ability to move their neck without much resistance. At the end of the treatment, the neck should again be given with gentle kneading, grasping and rolling. The twisting technique must be performed very carefully.

Notes and Suggestions

(1) Stiff necks are a common soft tissue injury. After a successful qigong acupressure therapy, patients should practice some physical exercise to maintain the positive therapeutic results.

(2) The above-mentioned twisting technique must be carefully performed to avoid any injury to the joints of cervical spinal vertebrae.

Case Report

Mr. Chen, a 56-year-old patient from Hebei Province, first visited a clinic in July 1976 because of a suddenly appeared pain of left shoulder and neck after getting up in that morning. In addition, he also suffered from stiffness, limited rotation and restricted forward and backward flexing of the neck. After 2 treatments of qigong acupressure therapy and application of external qi, the patient's sufferings were completely relieved.

Periarthritis of the Shoulder

Causes and Symptoms

Periarthritis of the shoulder is due to the aging process, deficiency of qi and blood, poor nutrition and invasion of wind, cold and damp evils. The main symptoms are gradually aggravated shoulder pain (severity is less during the day and worsen at night); marked limitation of shoulder joint movement, (making it difficult to raise the arm and put on clothes); and (at the late stages) atrophy of the shoulder muscles.

Techniques: Finger-pressing, palm-pressing, kneading, plucking, pinching, grasping, rotating, shaking and patting techniques with activated qi.

Treatment Procedure

(1) Patients take a sitting posture with the neck and shoulder relaxed. Stand beside the diseased side of the patient and knead and press the neck, shoulder and back with activated qi for 5-6 minutes and then pluck the medial border of the scapula, coracoid process and the long and short heads of the humeral biceps. The manipulating force applied should be gradually increased in intensity to reach deeper and deeper layers of the body. This technique is used to promote blood circulation, stop pain and facilitate joint movement.

(2) Gentle and slow pinching and grasping and kneading techniques are applied 6-12 times to the arm from its proximal end to the distal end. The arm is passively

moved, maximizing its range of forward flexion, backward extension and rotation until the patients can no longer tolerate the pain. Finally, rotating, shaking and patting techniques are applied to the shoulder.

Notes and Suggestions

(1) The therapeutic procedure should be carried out accurately and appropriately. For patients at early stages with severe pain, the manipulation should be gentle; for patients at late stages, the pressure and activated qi should be applied vigorously enough to reach deeply-located diseased part.

(2) Periarthritis of the shoulder should be carefully differentiated from acute afflictions, such as suppurative arthritis and tuberculosis of the shoulder joint; severe trauma, such as bone fracture and dislocation of the shoulder joint; and bone tumors. These serious diseases require special treatment.

(3) Patients should perform physical exercise to hasten the recovery of shoulder joint functioning. These following exercises are recommended: climbing a tree with fingers (6-12 times) to train the muscles of the shoulder and arm; rotating the arm over a wide range with the arm abducted and laterally stretched (6-12 turns); and the abducting and backward raising exercise 6-12 times) and the hand passively pulled to the normal side 6-12 times. Patients should perform the above exercises with a concentrated mind, keeping pace with their natural respiratory movement.

Case Report

Mrs. Wang, a 57-year-old cadre from Hebei Province, first visited a clinic in June 1978. For a half-year she experienced pain and limitation of movement in the left shoulder joint. The shoulder pain was aggravated when the patient was tired and her sleep was often interrupted at night. A physical examination showed that the patient had limited movement when she tried to raise her arm over her head or extend it backward. After ten qigong acupressure therapy sessions, the shoulder pain was relieved and the locomotive functions were almost completely recovered. The patient was asked to regularly carry on exercises to maintain her good therapeutic result.

Cervical Spondylopathy

Causes and Symptoms

Cervical spondylopathy, also called cervical spondylosis, is a syndrome due to degenerative change in the cervical vertebrae and compression and stimulation of the cervical nerve roots caused by many pathological processes, such as hypertrophic arthritis of the cervical spinal column, protrusion and degeneration of intervertebral discs, and functional disturbance of small joints of the cervical vertebrae. The predilection sites of the diseases are the 4th to 6th cervical vertebrae. The onset age of patients with this diesease is from 40 to 60 years old. The incidence of the disease is higher in men than in women and it is related to occupational strain due to the constant forward declination of the neck during work such as paper work, typewriting, sewing and embroidery.

At early stages, patients may suffer from a blunt or aching pain and accompanied with soreness, heaviness and swelling; at middle stages, pain may radiate to the back of the head, behind ears and eyes, neck, shoulder, back, chest, arm and even down to the forearm, hand; and at late stages, patients begin to show functional disturbance and muscular atrophy of the arm (for example, the arm can not be raised up and grasping power is reduced). In some patients with compression in the spinal cord, the functional disturbance and muscular atrophy may appear in the lower limbs: A CAT scan is necessary for these people.

A physical examination may show an increased muscular tension in the neck, shoulder and back with round or rod-like nodules in the muscles and tender spots beside the spinous and transverse processes of the involved cervical vertebrae. Movement in the neck tends to be limited; sometimes a clicking or cracking sound may accompany movement. In severe conditions, the neck may lose its natural curve and even assume a reverse curve and angulation. The muscles of the shoulder, scapula and arm may be atrophic with reduced muscular tension and strength, and the tendon reflexes may be reduced in extent and responsiveness. But in patients with spinal cord injury due to compression, muscular tension may be increased and the tendon reflexes may be exaggerated.

X-ray films may show hyperosteogeny of the anterior and posterior borders of the cervical vertebrae, especially common in the 4th and 5th intervertebral spaces, which may become narrowed; and the natural curvature may be lost and the spinal column may become straight or produce a reverse convexity.

A diagnosis can easily be made from symptoms, physical signs and X-ray findings, but it should be carefully differentiated from protrusion of the intervertebral disc, tuberculosis of the spinal column, scalenus syndrome, cervical rib and spinal cord diseases.

Techniques: Finger-pressing, palm-pressing, plucking and stretching techniques with activated qi.

Treatment Procedure

(1) Traction Applied to the Neck: Flex the elbow joint of one arm and use the palm to support the occiput of the patient; use another palm to support the chin, and then slowly raise the patient's head upward. For patients with pain of the stenoclei-domastoid muscle, use one hand to hold the occiput and use the thumb of the other hand to press tender spots with activated qi until the pain is relieved.

(2) Twisting the Neck: Because this is a rather dangerous manipulation, it must be done skillfully by a qualified qigong practioner after a correct diagnosis has been made. Use one palm to support and lift the cheek of the patient and use the other hand to press the spinous process of the subluxated vertebra. Gently turn the head to one side until it can turn no more. Use a sudden twist of small amplitude to produce sharp crack in the neck vertabrae.

(3) Finger-Pressing: If the irritative symptoms can not be relieved by above treatments and the pain is aggravated by cough, finger-pressing is applied to the

affected part and the patient is asked to cough. Pressure is applied when the patient coughs. It can release the compression of the nerve roots and relieve the irritative symptoms.

Notes and Suggestions

(1) The twisting must be carefully done to avoid any additional injury to the articulation of the cervical vertebrae.

(2) Cervical spondylopathy is a common disease and qigong acupressure can produce a good therapeutic effect, but regular physical exercise should also be practiced to maintain positive therapeutic results.

Case Report

Mr. Zhang, a 58-year-old retired worker from Hebei Province, had a 10-year history of neck pain, neck movement limitation and arm numbness. A physical examination showed an apparent tenderness beside the 6th and 7th cervical vertebrae and neck stiffness. Forward and backward flexion of the neck was restricted. X-ray films showed hyperosteogeny of the 5th to 7th cervical vertebrae with local calcification and slightly narrowed intervertebral spaces. After 6 treatments of qigong acupressure therapy (with application of external qi), the neck pain and limitation of movement was alleviated. After another course of 6 treatments, his sufferings were almost entirely relieved. The patient was asked to do regular physical exercise for his neck to maintain the therapeutic result.

Chest and Rib Pain

Causes and Symptoms:

The liver and gallbladder meridians pass through the flank region. Chest and rib pain is due to stagnation of liver qi, suppression of yang in the chest, excessiveness of internal cold (yin) evil, and stasis of qi and blood in the meridians. Also, chest pain may be aggravated by respiratory movement.

Diagnosis and Treatment

(1) Suppression of Chest Yang and Excessiveness of Internal Cold Evil:

Symptoms: Patients may suffer from chest pain, cough and shortness of breath.

Therapeutic Techniques: Pressing and kneading with activated qi over the 1st to 10th thoracic vertebrae 3-5 times and finger-pressing to the Yunmen (LU 2) and Huagai (RN 20) points.

Healing Effects: This treatment can adjust qi, move turbid waste product downward, dispel cold and promote flow of yang.

(2) Blood Stasis and Meridian Blockage:

Symptoms: The patients may suffer from stationary pricking pain in chest.

Therapeutic Techniques: Finger-pressing, palm-pressing, kneading and pushing tender spots 6-12 times.

Healing Effects: This treatment can remove blood stasis, promote blood circulation, release obstruction in the meridians and stop pain.

(3) Stagnation of Liver Qi and Deficiency of Essence and Blood:

Symptoms: Patients may suffer from high mental irritability and fury, pain and swelling in the chest, poor appetite and chest distress.

Therapeutic Technique: Pressing and kneading the lateral chest wall and ribs with activated qi and grasping the shoulder and back muscles.

Healing Effects: This treatment can relieve restriction of liver qi, adjust qi and stop pain.

Techniques

Besides the techniques mentioned in the above paragraphs of diagnosis and treatment, routine qigong acupressure therapy for the chest and abdomen may also be adopted to treat patients.

Treatment Procedure

Patients lie on their back with the body relaxed and the knee joints flexed. Qigong practioner stands beside the patient and applies routine qigong acupressure therapy on chest and abdomen.

Notes and Suggestions

(1) Although qigong acupressure therapy can expand the chest cavity and relieve chest pain, it should be carefully used to treat patients with emphysema or pleurisy and it is absolutely prohibited to use for patients with fractures or tumors of the ribs.

(2) The pressure used in qigong acupressure for chest and rib pain should be evenly, gently and flexibly applied with activated qi delivered through the fingers and palms.

Case Report

Mrs. Chen, a 55-year-old hospital worker, first visited a clinic in October 1986. For 2 years she suffered chest and rib pain due to unknown cause. She had seen a surgeon, but no organic pathological changes were found and no therapeutic effect could be obtained by physical therapy. A physical examination showed tenderness over the right chest between the 7th and 8th ribs. After qigong acupressure therapy was applied 6 times, her chest pain was reduced; after another 12 treatments all sufferings were almost completely relieved.

Stomachaches

Causes and Symptoms

The stomachache is due to injury of the spleen and stomach caused by attacks of adverse liver qi on the spleen after a lasting mental depression or repeated anger. Other causes include worrying and on inadequate diet regime followed over a long time. Diet problems can stem from an irregular food intake (either too full or too restricted), eating and drinking too much at one meal, or frequently eating too much spicy or cold food. In patients with deficiency and impaired function of spleen and stomach, food and drinks can not be digested well causing them to suffer from epigastric pain (stomachache) from the invasion of cold evil. Stomachaches may be either very severe with a prompt onset or dull in nature. Patients with coldness and deficiency in the spleen and stomach may suffer from abdominal fullness and swelling; and patients with stomachache due to attacks of adverse liver qi in the stomach may suffer from a wandering pain over the left and right hypochondriac region. The pain may be reduced after belching. Patients may also suffer from regurgitation of sour fluid, nausea, vomiting, diarrhea or constipation. Chronic patients may have dizziness, blurred vision, unstable sleep, lassitude and mental and physical tiredness.

Diagnosis and Treatment

(1) Stagnation of Liver Qi:

Symptoms: Patients may suffer from epigastric pain and swelling, radiating to bilateral ribs, regurgitation of sour fluid, bitter taste in the mouth and belching due to attacks of adverse liver qi on the spleen and stomach. The symptoms may be alleviated after breaking wind, but emotional upheavals may aggravate them.

Therapeutic Techniques: Rubbing and vibrating the painful area with activated qi and finger-pressing along the spinal column 6-12 times.

Healing Effects: The treatment can disperse liver qi, regulate stomach function and stop pain.

(2) Stagnation of Food in Stomach:

Symptoms: Patients may suffer from epigastric pain and swelling, nausea, vomiting and regurgitation of sour and foul vomit caused by taking too much food and drink in one meal and the stagnation of indigested food.

Therapeutic Techniques: Rubbing the epigastric region with activated qi and grasping and pinching along the Urinary Bladder Meridian 6-12 times.

Healing Effects: This treatment can promote the digestion of food, relieve stagnation of food, adjust circulation of qi and stop pain.

(3) Sinking of Spleen Qi Downward:

Symptoms: Patients may suffer from epigastric swelling (especially severe after meals), intestinal gurgles, gradually impaired appetite, wasting and weakness of body, dizziness, palpitation of heart, occasional constipation or diarrhea, and a feeling of heaviness of the stomach.

Therapeutic Techniques: Pushing, kneading, vibrating and pinching the back with activated qi.

Healing Effects: The treatment can tonify the spleen and stomach and replenish qi.

Techniques

Routine qigong acupressure therapy for chest and abdomen and finger-pressing, palm-pressing and kneading on tender spots.

Treatment Procedure

Patients lie on their back with the knee joints flexed. Stand by the right side of the patient and apply routine qigong acupressure therapy for the chest and abdomen; then, with the patients on their stomach and legs straight apply the finger-pressing technique with activated qi along the spinal column.

Notes and Suggestions

(1) In patients with serious complications of gastric peptic ulcer, such as the gastric hemorrhage or perforation, qigong acupressure may be applied at remote acupoints of the related meridians rather than at the local acupoints.

(2) Patients are better off eating more meals with less food than less meals with more food. Sour, spicy, raw and cold food should be avoided.

(3) Patients with ptosis of the stomach may use a girdle to support the stomach; they should also perform physical exercise like sit-ups and leg-lifts.

Case Report

Mrs. Chang, a 50-year-old cadre, first visited a clinic in October 1986 with a chief complaint of repeated attacks of stomachache, usually predisposed by tiredness or attacks of cold weather. The exacerbation of stomachache which urged her to visit this clinic was quickly stopped by a qigong acupressure therapy during which the patient obtained a hot sensation in her abdomen.

Abdominal Pain

Causes and Symptoms

As a common symptom, abdominal pain may appear in many diseases and it is usually evoked by weather extremes (too cold or too hot), inadequate food or disharmony between qi and blood.

Diagnosis and Treatment

(1) Abdominal Pain Due to Disturbance of Qi:

Symptoms: The patients may suffer from a wandering and fluctuated pain and abdominal swelling caused by emotional disturbance, attack of adverse liver qi to spleen and stomach, and qi stagnation.

Therapeutic Techniques: If abdominal pain can not be controlled by routine qigong acupressure therapy for chest and abdomen and pinching the mucles along the spine with activated qi, finger-pressing with activated qi may be applied at the bilateral Pishu (BL 20) and Zusanli (ST 36) points.

Healing Effects: The treatment can disperse liver qi, strengthen spleen, adjust circulation of qi and stop pain.

(2) Abdominal Pain Due to Blood Disturbances:

Symptoms: Due to stagnation of blood and disturbances in qi circulation, patients may suffer from stationary pain in the abdomen and thirst (without a desire to drink water).

Therapeutic Techniques: Rubbing around umbilicus and Dantian and finger-pressing with activated qi along the liver and spleen meridians from the medial part of abdomen downward to the medial malleolus 6-12 times.

Healing Effects: This treatment can remove blood stasis, promote blood circulation, release meridian blockages and stop pain.

(3) Abdominal Pain Caused by Cold Evil:

Symptoms: Due to deficiency of qi in spleen and stomach and repeated attacks of cold evil caused by intake of raw and cold food, patients may suffer from a dull, lingering pain in the abdomen and diarrhea. The abdominal pain can be alleviated by warmth and the application of pressure.

Therapeutic Techniques: Rubbing with activated qi around the umbilicus for 5-6 minutes.

Healing Effects: This treatment can warm up the stomach, promote digestion of food, dispel cold evil and stop pain.

(4) Abdominal Pain Caused by Heat Evil:

Symptoms: Patients may suffer from abdominal pain caused by intake of too much greasy food or alcohol and accumulation of heat evil in the stomach and intestines, so that they are afraid of the application of pressure to their abdomen. Patients may also suffer from poor appetite, belching (with foul odors) and diarrhea or constipation.

Therapeutic Techniques: Palm-pressing and kneading lumbar spinal column with activated qi, finger-pressing at Changqiang (DU 1), or rotational rubbing over the lower abdomen and pressing from the thigh downward along the Foot-Yangming Meridian. Repeat 6-12 times.

Healing Effects: This treatment can clear heat evil, relieve qi blockages, evacuate stagnated food, and stop pain.

Techniques

Pushing, kneading, rubbing and erasing with activated qi and routine qigong acupressure therapy for chest and abdomen as well as therapeutic methods mentioned in above diagnosis and treatment paragraphs.

Treatment Procedure

Patients take a supine posture with their knee joints flexed. Stand beside the patient and put the central part of the right palm over the patient's umbilicus; overlap the right hand with the left hand and quickly but gently rub, press and knead the abdomen (in a clockwise direction) with activated qi 6-12 times; and then to gently push and rub the abdomen on both sides and to umbilicus with activated qi until hot sensation and intestinal gurgles are produced in the abdomen.

Notes and Suggestions

(1) The therapeutic effect of qigong acupressure therapy for abdominal pain is very satisfactory, but for patients with acute conditions, the clinical progression of the disease should be carefully watched.

(2) The palm should be warmed up by activated qi before it is used to perform the rotational rubbing to expel wind, relieve distension and stagnation, remove meridian blockages and stop pain.

Case Report

Wang, a 16-year-old sportsman, first visited a clinic in December 1985 with a chief complaint of repeated attacks of abdominal pain caused by exhaustive physical training and by attacks of coldness. His severe abdominal pain caused disturbance in sleep, food intake and participation in sports. Besides a sallow complexion and a weak body, the physical examination did not show other abnormality. Abdominal pain was alleviated after three qigong acupressure therapy treatments (with application of external qi); all sufferings were almost completely relieved after 6 treatments. Advice was given to the patient to carefully control his food intake and avoid physical exhaustion.

Constipation

Causes and Symptoms

Constipation is difficulty with and/or prolonged interval of defecation. In general, the transit time of mixed food in the digestive canal of human beings takes 20-40 hours. The postponement of defecation over 2 days is considered constipation, although some normal persons may have a regular defecation every 2-3 days. Common causes of constipation are: addiction to alcohol, eating too much spicy, hot and greasy food, deficiency of body fluid after febrile diseases (with dryness and heat evils retained in intestines); excessive worrying, emotional depression, sitting on chairs over a long time without sufficient physical activity and circulation of qi; and a weak and lean physique after chronic diseases, delivery of a baby, or a deficiency of both qi and blood (mostly in aged people). A deficiency of qi may reduce the motility of the intestines to transport waste products of food and deficiency of blood and body fluid, which moistens and lubricates the intestines to facilitate the passage of stools. Constipated patients may have a bowel movement every 3-5 days or 6-7 days and even over a longer time, and the stool may be very dry, hard and difficult to pass; but in some patients, even though the stools are not very dry and hard, they can not entirely pass. Patients may also suffer from headaches, dizziness, chest distress, abdominal swelling, belching, impairment of appetite, unstable sleep and annoyance and are easy to get angry. There may also be some complications, such as hemorrhoids and anal fissure.

Techniques

Finger-pressing, palm-pressing, pushing, rubbing and vibrating with activated qi.

Treatment Procedure

(1) Patients take a supine posture. Apply finger-pressing with activated qi at the Daheng (SP 15), Qihai (RN 6) and Guanyuan (RN 4) points; palm-pressing, pushing, vibrating and rubbing over the abdomen to produce a hot sensation in the abdomen and increase peristalsis in the intestines.

(2) Patients lie on their stomach. Apply pressing and pushing with activated qi to the Dachangshu (BL 25), Xiaochangshu (BL 27), Baliao (BL 30-33) and Changqiang (DU 1) points and pinching the muscles along the spine to produce a hot sensation in the abdomen and increased intestinal peristalsis. Repeat 6-12 times.

(3) Patients take a sitting posture. Use the palm to horizontally push and knead the patient's back beside the spinal column from its upper part downward over the Dachangshu and Xiaochangshu points to produce a hot sensation in the abdomen. Repeat 6-12 times.

Notes and Suggestions

(1) Besides regular treatments received in clinics, patients should do physical exercise and self-treatment with rubbing and kneading over the abdomen 2-3 times a day to promote intestinal peristalsis.

(2) Patients should eat more fruits and vegetables and should keep away from the spicy food.

(3) Complications of hemorrhoids and anal fissures should be treated by surgical intervention.

Case Report

Mrs. Li, a 62-year-old housewife, first visited a clinic in May 1986. For 10 years she had suffered from constipation. The patient usually passed stools (accompanied with abdominal pain, dizziness, headaches and restlessness) once every 2-3 days. The constipation could not be corrected by drugs. The constipation and abdominal pain was slightly alleviated after 6 treatments of qigong acupressure therapy (with application of external qi); the condition was almost completely relieved after another 12 treatments. The patient was asked to regularly perform health maintenance exercises for the abdomen to enhance the motility of the stomach and intestines.

Heat Stroke

Causes and Symptoms

Heat stroke is a disease with high fever, a disturbance of water and electrolyte metabolism, circulatory failure and impairment of nervous adjustment of body temperature. It is caused by thermal irradiation due to an environment of high temperature or exposed, scorching sunlight. There are two disposing factors: aged people and children, chronic patients with very weak physiques, and pregnant women are most susceptible to heat stroke; and heat stroke usually appears in extremely hot seasons under scorching sunshine and in an unbroken spell of hot, humid weather. Heat strokes may be divided into three varieties:

(1) Sun Stroke: Patients may suffer from severe headaches, dizziness and tinnitus due to brain damage caused by the exposure of the head to scorching sunlight. Severe cases may develop restlessness and the symptoms of respiratory and peripheral circulatory failure, and the body temperature is not necessarily very high.

(2) Heat Stroke: Patients may suffer from an extremely high body temperature (as high as 40-42 degrees centigrade); dry, hot and cyanotic skin; and mental confusion or coma due to accumulation of too much heat energy in the body.

(3) Heat Cramps: Patients may suffer from muscular aching and cramps, especially common in the muscle of abdomen and the four limbs, which are caused by profuse sweating and loss of large amount of sodium compounds. One-third of the total patients experience cramps. Generally, patients are mentally clear.

Techniques

Finger-pressing, palm-pressing and pinching the muscles along the spine with activated qi.

Treatment Procedure

(1) Finger-Pressing and Daoyin Qi: First pinch the nail beds of the patient with activated qi; press Hegu (LI 4) and Renzhong (DU 26) with the finger and then Daoyin qi into the patient's head to spread it all over the body and adjust the function of the nervous system.

(2) Palm-Pressing and Pinching: Patients lie on their stomach or on the side of their body. Use the finger and palm to press the Du Meridian up and down and pinching the muscles along the spine to promote blood circulation through the Du and urinary bladder meridians. Repeat 6-12 times.

Notes and Suggestions

(1) Heat stroke patients should be moved immediately to a cool place to inhale fresh air; this will enrich the supply of oxygen to the brain tissues.

(2) Cold drinks should be supplied to patients to provide more fluids and nutrients to improve metabolism.

(3) Patients should have a good rest after they have recovered from this critical condition.

Case Report

Mr. Lin, a 58-year-old farmer from Hebei Province, first visited a clinic in July 1978 with a complaint of headaches, dizziness, tinnitus and annoyance caused by exhausting farm work on a very hot, sunny day. The patient had no fever and was mentally clear. He suffered from profuse sweating over the body and muscular pain in the shoulder, back and limbs. After a physical examination, a diagnosis of heat stroke was made; after qigong acupressure therapy and application of external qi, all sufferings were completely relieved.

Dysmenorrhea

Causes and Symptoms

From the viewpoint of traditional Chinese medicine, body resistance is reduced during the menstrual period and women are more susceptible to the attack of external evils and injury from emotional disturbances. Mental depression may injure liver and cause stagnation of qi; and blood; and the invasion of cold evil into the Chong (thoroughfare) and Ren (conception) meridians may also cause stagnation and coagulation of blood, which may in turn cause deficiency of qi and blood and poor nourishment of the uterus. Therefore, the stagnation of qi and blood is the basic cause of dysmenorrhea.

According to Western medicine, dysmenorrhea is related to mental stress, emotional unstability, mental depression and fright; or it can be due to diseases of the ovary, uterus or endocrine glands. Menstrual pain may appear 1-2 days before the onset of the menstrual period until the start of menstrual flow and it may last from just a few hours to 1 or 2 days. The pain is spastic or dull in nature; other symptons include a pale complexion, cold sweating, cold limbs, nausea, vomiting, and even syncope in severe cases. In general, menstrual pain is located in the lower abdomen and in severe cases it may radiate to the lower back, anterior and medical sides of the thigh and even to the knee and posterior side of the leg. Dysmenorrhea may spontaneously stop after marriage and childbirth.

Techniques

Finger-Pressing, palm-pressing, and rotatory rubbing with activated qi.

Treatment Procedure

(1) Finger-Pressing: Patients take a supine posture with the body relaxed. Stand beside the patient and gently press the tender spots of the abdominal wall with the finger to produce a hot sensation in the abdomen and lower limbs; then press the Guanyuan (RN 4), Qizhong (RN 8), Qipang (EX point, beside umbilicus) and Qihai (RN 6) points.

(2) Rotational Rubbing (or vibrating): Patients lie face down. Stand beside the patient and use the palm with activated qi to press Yaoyan (EX-B7) and acupoints on the buttocks, such as Shenshu (BL 23), Pangguangshu (BL 28) and Baliao (BL 30-33); then apply vibration with activated qi to produce a hot sensation in the abdomen. At the same time, acupressure is applied to the bilateral Zusanli (ST 36), Yanglingquan (GB 34) and Sanyinjiao (SP 6) points.

Notes and Suggestions

(1) Throughout the therapeutic course, patients should rest and avoid physical exertion.

(2) Patients not eat cold and raw food or take cold water showers; they should also protect themselves from cold and damp weather.

(3) Patients should also minimize the causal factors such as nervousness, terror and anxiety.

Case Report

Mrs. Liu, a 40-year-old medical staff of a hospital, first visited a clinic in October 1986 with a complaint of lower abdominal, lumbar and sacral pain, and heaviness which was exacerbated during the menstrual period. A lump was detected in the lower abdomen by physical examination and it was identified by ultrasonic examination as a hysteromyoma. After 24 treatments of qigong acupressure therapy with applicaion of external qi, the abdominal pain was relieved; the disappearance of the lump was verified by a follow-up ultrasonic examination.

Paralysis

Causes and Symptoms

Wei-syndrome in traditional Chinese medicine is characterized by weakness, immovability and muscular atrophy of the limbs. The same symptoms are found in multiple neuritis, sequela of poliomyelitis, early stages of acute myelitis, myasthenia gravis, chlorotic paralysis and peripheral paralysis in Western medicine. The main symptoms of Wei-syndrome are weakness and flaccidness of muscles and loss of locomotive function. At the early stages, patients may have fevers; after that weakness and partial paralysis of the upper and lower (left or right) limbs appears and gradually worsens until complete paralysis develops. The muscles may gradually and painlessly become atrophied.

Diagnosis and Treatment

(1) Damp-Heat Type:

Symptoms: Besides progressive paralysis due to damage of the Yangming Meridian (caused by damp-heat) which may disturb the locomotive function of muscles and joints, patients may also suffer from heaviness of the body, turbid urine and a hot sensation in their feet.

Therapeutic Techniques: Routine qigong acupressure therapy for the chest and abdomen is applied first to adjust the spleen and stomach and then grasping with activated qi is applied along the medial and lateral sides of lower limbs to the ankle joints. Repeat 6-12 times.

Healing Effects: The treatment can clear damp-heat and promote the circulation of qi and blood.

(2) Heat Evil in the Lungs:

Symptoms: Patients may suffer from fever, cough, thirst and scanty, dark urine in addition to progressive muscular paralysis caused by the invasion of wind and heat evils into the lungs. This condition consumes and reduces the body fluid of lungs, leaving an insuffient amount to nourish and moisten the muscles and blood vessels.

Therapeutic Techniques: Pinching the muscles along the spine and gently rubbing the lumbar and sacral region along the Urinary Bladder Meridian down to the lower limbs and finger-pressing, pinching, patting and pulling-toe with activated qi. Repeat 4-6 times.

Healing Effects: The treatment can clear heat evil in lungs and nourish muscles and tendons.

(3) Deficiency of Liver and Kidney:

Symptoms: Patients may suffer from soreness and weakness in the back and loins, weakness of the lower limbs, emission, premature ejaculation of semen, dizziness and blurred vision due to deficiency of essence, and poor nutrition of the muscles and blood vessels resulting from a chronic consuming disease or frequent sexual activities.

Therapeutic Techniques: Pressing and kneading techniques with activated qi applied to the acupoints on the back along the gallbladder meridian down to the ankle joints.

Healing Effects: This treatment can disperse liver, tonify kidney and nourish muscles and tendons.

Techniques

Pushing, kneading, pinching, grasping, finger-pressing, palm-pressing and Daoyin with activated qi may also be adopted besides the therapeutic methods mentioned above.

Treatment Procedure

(1) Routine qigong acupressure therapy selected according to the differential diagnosis of a syndrome is applied with adequate strength.

(2) Patients take a supine posture. Put your palm over the Baihui (DU 20) point

on the head of the patient and apply qigong acupressure therapy and Daoyin qi into the body to release meridian blockages.

(3) Patients lie face down. Push the back of the patient along the lines beside the spinal column (Du Meridian) and press and knead the back with activated qi up and down repeatedly. This will relax the muscles. Then grasp, press and knead the involved limbs to promote blood circulation.

Notes and Suggestions

Qigong acupressure therapy for chronic paralytic patients must be regularly and persistently applied over a long time to obtain a satisfactory result; at the same time patients should do physical exercise and receive some other necessary treatment to maintain the therapeutic result.

Case Report

King, a 14-year-old boy, was brought to a clinic to treat left cerebral palsy and sequelae of poliomyelitis which he had suffered for over 10 years. He had mild muscular atrophy in the right lower limb, impaired ability to walk, weakness on the right side of the body, and a reduction of circumference of the right thigh by 1-2 cm with a 3-4 grade of myodynamia. After 12 treatments of qigong acupressure with external qi, the circumference of the diseased leg was increased by about 1 cm, the weakness of the right side of the body was alleviated and his gait was improved.

Emission

Causes and Symptoms

Emission may be divided into two types: with or without sexual dreams. Abnormal ejaculation of semen is due to excessiveness of premier fire or sexual desire, stirring up of heart yang or kidney yang, overfatigue or by too much worry and disharmony between heart and kidney. Besides spontaneous ejaculation of semen during dreams about sexual activity, patients may suffer from dizziness, vertigo, lassitude, tinnitus and soreness of the lower back. If this condition lasts over a long period of time, patients may have spontaneous ejaculation of semen without dreams, and it may happen even during the day time without sexual impulses. Typical patients are very weak and lean, and they may also suffer from palpitation of the heart and impotence.

Techniques

Finger-pressing, palm-pressing, pinching and patting with activated qi.

Treatment Procedure

(1) Finger-Pressing: Patients take a supine posture. Apply finger-pressing with activated qi at the Sanyinjiao (SP 6), Yangjiao (GB 35), Pishu (BL 20), Sanjiaoshu (BL 22) and Mingmen (DU 4) points. Repeat 3-5 times. For patients having emissions without dreams, finger-pressing may be applied at the Shenshu (BL 23), Mingmen (DU 4), Qugu (RN 2) and Baliao (BL 30-33) points together with the patting technique at Baliao (BL 30-33) until a hot sensation can be felt around the acupoints.

(2) Pinching: Patients take a supine posture. Pinch the base of the nails and toe

nails and the phalangeal joints of toes with activated qi 3-5 times until a hot sensation can be felt.

(3) Patting: Patting with activated qi is applied over the umbilical region or lower abdomen until a hot sensation can be felt over the perineal region.

(4) Physical Exercise: Patients may do the Robust Man Squatting and Standing-Up exercise and the patting exercise at lower Dantian every day until a hot sensation can be felt in the abdomen. To maintain a sound sleep, patients should try their best to release mental stress and nervousness. They should lie on their side to sleep.

Case Report

Mr. Wang, a 42-year-old man from Heilongjiang Province, first visited a clinic in May 1986 with complaints of dizziness, vertigo, tinnitus, lassitude, soreness and pain in the back and loins, noctural emissions with dreams, impotence, palpitation of the heart and general weakness of the body. His face was dark blue in color. The urogenital examination did not show any abnormality. After qigong acupressure therapy and application of external qi 6 times, the symptoms were apparently alleviated and after another 6 treatments the emission was almost completely controlled.

Impotence

Causes and Symptoms

Impotence is a symptom of sexual disorder characterized by a failed or reduced penis erection that is not strong enough for sexual intercourse. It is secondary to some chronic wasting diseases or caused by too frequent sexual activity or excessive masturbation. According to traditional Chinese medical theory, the cause of impotence is the deficiency of kidney qi, declination of the source of vitality and exhaustion of essence or damage to the kidney.

Techniques

Routine qigong acupressure therapy for the chest and abdomen may be adopted to treat impotence.

Treatment Procedure

(1) Palm-Pressing: Patients take a supine posture. Press their lower abdomen with the palm and activated qi from the umbilicus down to Qugu (RN 2) 6-12 times with a gentle pressure at the beginning, gradually increased to enhance kidney and Dantian qi.

(2) Patting: Patients lie on their back and then on their abdomen. Pat the lower abdomen and then the lumbar and sacral region [Baliao (BL 30-33)] with the palm and activated qi 6-12 times to produce a hot sensation.

(3) Physical Exercise: Patients may perform the Robust Man Squatting and Standing-Up exercise or pat their own lower abdomen in a lying posture. The mind should be concentrated at the posterior Dantian to enhance kidney and spleen qi.

Case Report

Mr. Wu, a 53-year-old overseas Chinese from Indonnesia, first visited a clinic in

August 1985. He had been suffering from impotence for 5 years. He also suffered from constant dizziness, blurred vision, lassitude, soreness and weakness in the lower back and lower limbs, general weakness of the body and pale complexion. The urogenital examination did not show any abnormality. After 12 treatments of qigong acupressure therapy with application of external qi, his sufferings were much alleviated.

Mastitis

Causes and Symptoms Mastitis is a postpartum disease of the breast, more common in primipara, which is correspondent to mastitis in modern medicine. At the early stages, patients may suffer from redness, swelling and breast pain (often with lumps), reduced or obstructed milk ejection. General symptoms include chills, fever, nausea and severe thirst. When mammary abscesses are formed the breast are enlarged in size, raw red in color and throbbing with pain. At late stages, abscess may rupture if no prior treatment has been received; this is very difficult to heal. In traditional Chinese medicine, mastitis caused by the invasion of fire evil into the breast. This blocks the vessels and branches preventing the discharge of milk.

Techniques
Finger-pressing, finger-kneading, pushing, grasping, rubbing and vibrating with activated qi. This treatment can release blood stasis, promote blood circulation, increase milk discharge, control inflammation and stop pain. At early stages, the inflammation can be controlled by 3-5 treatments.

Treatment Procedure
(1) Patients take a sitting posture. Gently rub their chest with the proximal part of the palm using activated qi, pressing Rugen (ST 18) with the finger and then to push with the finger along the Yangming Meridian 6-12 times.

(2) Vibrating is applied with the center of the palm [inner Laogong (PC 8)] from the lumps of breast to the nipple to soften and resolve the lumps until a hot sensation is felt.

(3) Pinching and grasping with activated qi are applied to the scapular muscles and the patient's arm is pulled downward as your fist is used to push the axillary pit. This promotes milk discharge and produces a releasing sensation.

Case Report
Mrs. Cui, 28-year-old, first visited a clinic in March 1982 with a chief complaint of pain and distension in both breasts, which had lasted for 5 days. Besides red, swollen and tender lumps in both breasts, detected by palpation and the blockage of milk ejection, the patient also suffered from headaches, nausea and severe thirst. After qigong acupressure therapy and application of external qi 6 times, her symptoms were completely relieved.

Intestinal Obstructions

Causes and Symptoms
In traditional Chinese medicine the intestine is considered an organ for transpor-

tation of food materials. Obstruction of the intestine is a pathological condition, usually caused by impairment of its transporting function or blockage of qi and blood. In Western medicine, it can be divided into the simple and strangulated types. Simple intestinal obstruction can be cured by qigong acupressure therapy. Patients with simple intestinal obstruction may suffer from paroxysmal abdominal colic with high-pitched intestinal gurgles, repeated vomiting (throwing out yellowish-green fluid or foul fluid with fecal material), abdominal distension, and occasional appearance of visible intestinal peristalsis. No wind or stools are passed.

Techniques

Besides routine qigong acupressure therapy for the chest and abdomen, finger-pressing, kneading, rubbing on the abdomen and pinching the muscles along the spine are also used to treat this disease. As mentioned in traditional Chinese medicine texts, "this pain is caused by obstruction and can be relieved if the blockage can be removed." Qigong acupressure can promote stomach and intestinal peristalsis, help the passing of wind, reduce abdominal swelling, alleviate or release intestinal obstruction, the discharge stagnated intestinal content, adjust intestinal function and stop pain.

Treatment Procedure

(1) Patients take a supine posture. First apply routine qigong acupressure therapy for the chest and abdomen with gentle and smooth kneading and rubbing maneuvers (6-12 times) and then to apply the finger-pressing maneuver along stomach meridian to Zusanli until the intestinal flatus can be passed.

(2) Patients lie on their stomach. Knead the Du Meridian first and then apply the Nieji maneuver with the even-reinforcing and even-reducing technique to promote circulation of qi and blood, remove blood stasis and stop pain.

Case Report

Mr. Cheng, a 55-year-old man from Hebei Province, first visited a clinic in June 1978 with a complaint of paroxysmal abdominal colic and repeated vomiting. This had been going on for 5 days. Six months before the onset of the abdominal pain, he underwent an abdominal operation followed by a surgical complication of intestinal obstruction. A physical examination showed abdominal swelling and tenderness with a high-pitched intestinal gurgling sound. After 10 treatments of qigong acupressure therapy with application of external qi (2-3 times a day), his symptoms were almost completely relieved.

Diabetes Mellitus

Causes and Symptoms

As mentioned in traditional Chinese medical literature, diabetes mellitus is caused by disturbances in stomach and spleen function and accumulation of heat evil in the body due to eating too much sweet and greasy food and drinking too much alcohol. In Western medicine it is included in metabolic diseases and caused by pathogenic factors related to mental activity, environment, diet, obesity, alcohol consumption, and sexual activity. Common clinical manifestations of diabetes are diuresis, thirst (with a desire to drink too much water) overeating, fatigue, pathologic leanness, occasional ketoacidosis; also found are serious complications of the heart, brain, kidney, microcirculatory system, liver and gallbladder, nervous system and skin, as well as severe infections in the body. Laboratory examinations usually show hyperglycemia and positive urine sugar.

Techniques

Finger-pressing, palm-pressing, vibrating, kneading and with activated qi and pinching the muscles along the spine.

Treatment Procedure

(1) The patients take a supine posture. Use the thumb and middle finger of one hand to press Tianshu (ST 25) and Danzhong (RN 17) with activated qi and at the same time use a finger of another hand to press Yinlingquan (SP 9) with vibration for 3-5 minutes and then use one hand to press, push and knead the Qihai (RN 6), Yinjiao (RN 7) and Guanyuan (RN 4) points while the other hand presses the Sanyinjiao (SP 6), Shangwan (RN 13), Zhongwan (RN 12) and Jianli (RN 11) points with vibration; and finally, press and knead Zusanli (ST 36) with a finger and push and knead Liangmen (ST 21) with activated qi.

(2) Patients take a supine posture. Press and knead Zhangmen (LR 13) and use a finger of the other hand to press Jianjin (GB 21) with activated qi, and then press and knead the Zusanli (ST 36) and Neiguan (PC 6) points.

(3) Patients lie face down. Use the thumbs of both hands to press and knead the bilateral Feishu (BL 13) points with activated qi for 3-5 minutes. Then use both palms with activated qi delivered from the inner Laogong (PC 8) point to press and knead the Pishu (BL 20), Weishu (BL 21) and Shenshu (BL 23) points for 3-5 minutes; and finally, pinching the muscles along the spine 6-12 times.

Notes and Suggestions

(1) The even-reinforcing and even-reducing technique is used to strengthen the spleen and stomach, adjust liver qi and tonify yin of lungs, stomach and kidney (which has been consumed by heat evil). It also helps adjust and enhance the digestive and distributing function and improve the metabolism of the body.

(2) Qigong acupressure therapy can correct disturbed metabolism of carbohydrates, promote the regeneration and secretion of pancreatic islet cells, prevent complications and reduce the mortality of diabetes mellitus.

Case Report

Mrs. Li, a 48-year-old physician from Shanxi Province, first visited a clinic in 1984 with a history of diabetes mellitus for 10 years and symptoms of diuresis, thirst, overeating, tiredness and pathological leanness (all these symptoms had deteriorated in the recent half-year). She also had occasional attacks of ketoacidosis. The fast blood sugar was 150 mg% and the urine sugar was 3+. After qigong acupressure therapy and application of external qi 12 times, the urine sugar was reduced to 1+ and the fasting sugar to 125 mg%. Also, her general weakness was much improved.

Lumbago

Causes and Symptoms

Lumbago is a common symptom of many diseases, such as acute muscular sprain or chronic muscular strain of the lower back, fasciitis of the back and waist, prolapse of the lumbar intervertebral disc, etc. Patients may suffer from lumbago with pain radiating to the lower limb and aggravated by changes of weather; the movement of the waist may be markedly limited; and, the local diseased area may be tender and swollen. The causes of lumbago as mentioned by traditional physicians are wind and dampness evils, deficiency of kidney or acute sprain.

Diagnosis and Treatment

(1) Lumbago Due to Wind and Dampness Evils:

Symptoms: Lumbago caused by attacks of wind and dampness evils manifests as sore pain. It is aggravated on overcast and rainy days.

Therapeutic Techniques: Use the palm with activated qi to press and rub the posterior side of the thigh along the Urinary Bladder Meridian to the heel; also rub the loins with vibration until a hot and relaxing sensation can be felt by the patient.

Healing Effects: This treatment can dispel wind evil, discharge dampness evil, eliminate cold evil and stop pain.

(2) Lumbago Due to Deficiency of the Kidney:

Symptoms: A kidney essence deficiency can cause, in addition to lumbago, noctural emission, night sweating, and dizziness, tinnitus, soreness and weakness in the limbs.

Therapeutic Techniques: Kneading and pressing with activated qi are applied on the 1st to 5th lumbar vertebrae and along the three Yin Meridians of the Foot over the medial surface of the leg down to medial malleolus. Repeat 6-12 times.

Healing Effects: This treatment can tonify kidney, strengthen loins and enrich yin and yang.

(3) Lumbago Due to Acute Sprain:

Symptoms: Pain in lumbar region and limitation of movement may suddenly appear after falling down or after violent exercise. Patients usually assume an abnormal posture.

Therapeutic Techniques: Pinching and kneading with activated qi are applied to the lumbar muscles 6-12 times, followed by finger-pressing and strumming the back of the knee and Chengshan (BL 57) to release muscular spasms and stop pain.

Healing Effects: This treatment can promote blood circulation, remove blood stasis, release muscular spasms and stop pain.

Techniques

Besides the therapeutic methods mentioned in above paragraph on diagnosis and treatment, routine qigong acupressure therapy for the back and waist can also be adopted to treat lumbago.

Treatment Procedure

Patients lie on the stomach with both arms flexed and placed flat above the shoulders; their chest and abdomen and ankles are cushioned with pillows. Use the palm with activated qi to press and rub from Dazhui (DU 14) along the Du Meridian down to Mingmen (DU 4) or Baliao (BL 30-33) and then rub with activated qi and vibration along the Urinary Bladder Meridian from the upper part of thigh downward. Repeat 6-12 times.

Notes and Suggestions

(1) For patients with acute muscular sprain, X-rays should be taken to rule out bone fracture, tuberculosis and bone tumors before starting qigong acupressure therapy, because it is contraindicated to those diseases.

(2) Patients should take adequate rest throughout the therapeutic course and, when treatment ends, should start physical exercise to maintain the therapeutic effect of qigong acupressure therapy.

Case Report

Mr. Chen, a 28-year-old worker from Tianjin, first visited a clinic in October 1986 with a 1-year history of lumbago. The pain in the lower back was dull and sore in nature and aggravated after tiredness. Treatment with drugs had not produced any apparent therapeutic effect. After qigong acupressure therapy and application of external qi 6 times, the symptoms were markedly alleviated and after another 4 treatments, the lumbago was almost completely relieved.

Rheumatoid Arthritis

Causes and Symptoms

This is a chronic multiple arthropathy and can be divided into the peripheral (the four limbs) and central (spinal column, i.e. rheumatoid spondilitis or ankylosing spondilitis) types.

The cause of this disease is still unknown, but patients often complain of the pernicious influence of coldness and surgical trauma. The joints are often symmetrically and alternately involved, usually starting from the cervical vertebrae, fingers or iliosacral joint and gradually spreading to the large joints. Before the onset of the disease, patients may have some preliminary symptoms, such as the general weakness, lassitude, impaired appetite, spontaneous or night sweating, hypotension, loss of body weight, low fever or, in women, menstrual disturbance.

The symptoms of the early and late stages are varied:

(1) Early Stages: Arthralgia and local swelling usually starts from the small joints of the fingers and toes, wrist and ankle or from the iliosacral joint and spread upward to the lumbar, thoracic and cervical vertebrae. Several weeks or months later, patients may feel local tenderness and inflexibility in the joints with some clicking and cracking sounds. Arthralgia is worse at night and the worst in the morning; it may alleviated with gentle exercise.

(2) Late Stages: The joint movement is markedly limited and patients can have deformity in the joints, bone stiffness, muscular atrophy and paralysis. The upper limbs, the phalangeal and carpal joints of the patients may become rigid and deviated

to the ulnar side, the fingers may become deformed and (with their movements restricted), and the elbow and shoulder joints may be also affected; the lower limbs, the ankle, knee and hip joints of the patients may become rigid and their movements hindered. If arthritis occurs on the spinal column it may cause kyphotic deformity and dyspnea, and neck movements may be markedly restricted. A sudden backward flexing of the neck may cause a sudden death in patients with rigid, forward-bending neck deformity.

Diagnosis and Treatment

(1) Peripheral Type:

Techniques: Routine qigong acupressure therapy for the limbs and pushing, grasping, finger-pressing and stretching with activated qi.

Treatment Procedure:

Pushing and Grasping: Patients lie on their stomach. Push and grasp the buttocks with activated qi and then work downward through the hip and knee joints, as well as the posterior part of leg, to the ankle and toes. At the same time, use stretching on the lower limb until a hot sensation is produced in the patient.

Palm-Pressing: Patients sit on a stool. Press the medial and lateral sides of their arm with the palms from the shoulder down to the wrist 6-12 times; for patients with limitation of joint movement, vibrating with passive extending and flexing movement may be applied for 10 minutes.

Stretching: Patients take a supine posture. Use pressing and grasping first to relax the muscles of the lower limb and then to laterally rotate and abduct the lower limb and flex and extend the ankle joint inside and outside. Traction is applied to the hip, knee and ankle joints to promote blood circulation until a hot sensation can be detected in the diseased limb.

(2) Central Type:

Techniques: Routine qigong acupressure therapy for the back and the pushing, vibrating, pressing, rubbing and finger-pressing with activated qi.

Treatment Procedure:

Pushing and Vibrating: Patients take a sitting posture. Use the palm to push the lateral side of the neck and shoulder with vibration as the patients keep their head turned to the side and bending backward. Repeat until they feel a hot sensation in their neck.

Pressing and Grasping: Patients lie on their stomach. Repeatedly apply the pressing and grasping with vibration along the lines lateral to the spinal column from the level of Dazhui (DU 14) to the level of Mingmen (DU 4) to restore the patency of the Du and Urinary Bladder meridians.

Finger-Pressing: Patients lie on their stomach. Apply the finger-pressing with activated qi along the lines lateral to the spinal column from the level of Dazhui (DU 14) to the level of Baliao (BL 30-33) and then downward through the lower limb to Yongquan (KI 1). Repeat 6-12 times alone or combine it with the flat pushing 6-12 times.

Notes and Suggestions

(1) Patients are asked to do qigong exercise to improve their body resistance, but they should avoid overfatigue from too much vigorous physical exercise or too frequent sexual activity. Patients should also improve their diet and to keep their body warm.

(2) Rheumatoid arthritis is a chronic, stubborn disease, but movement in the involved joints can be restored or almost restored if the treatment is started in the early stages of the disease and the patients persistently practise the physical exercises for functional recovery. However, in late stages of this disease the treatment can only control the progression of the disease and alleviate local symptoms; and locomotive function can only be gradually improved through physical exercise over a long period of time.

(3) Qigong acupressure therapy can be applied to people over 60 years of age, but always after taking X-rays to rule out remarkable osteoporosis. For patients with osteoporosis, stretching and traction techniques, as well as sudden forward flexing of the neck are absolutely prohibited.

Case Report

Mr. Chen, 61-year-old, first visited a clinic in August 1978 with a 10-year history of rheumatoid arthritis in the finger, knee and hip joints and an exacerbation of the pain in the recent half-year. The patient suffered from general aching and stiffness of the back and waist. A physical examination showed limitation of movement in the four limbs and waist. Qigong acupressure therapy with application of external qi was applied once a day for 12 days. Each time the qigong acupressure treatment first produced a cool and then a warm sensation over the body together with an automatic movement of the limbs. After a course of 12 treatments, the patient felt much more relaxed in his body and flexible in his limbs and the sufferings were apparently alleviated. After another 24 treatments the arthralgia was almost completely relieved and the locomotive function of his body was nearly normal.

Calf Muscle Spasms

Causes and Symptoms

Calf muscle spasms are usually caused by overfatigue, such as by long-distance walking or swimming or due to exposure to coldness at night, such as when sleeping outside. Patients may suffer from immobility in the leg, intolerable spastic pain, inability to stand straight and stretching pain radiating to the ankle joint and toes.

Techniques

Patting, grasping, pressing, kneading and finger-pressing with activated qi.

Treatment Procedure

(1) Patting: Patients take a supine or sitting posture. Pat the leg of the patient with your palm, using adequate force and activated qi. This helps relieve muscular spasms.

(2) Pressing: The finger with activated qi is used to press the acupoints of the

urinary bladder meridian from the buttocks to the heel 3-6 times. This helps release meridian blockages, relieve muscular spasms and stop pain.

(3) Pinching and Grasping: Spastic calf muscles are pinched and grasped with the palm using activated qi from the top to the bottom of leg 6-12 times. This helps promote blood circulation, remove blood stasis, relieve muscular spasms and stop pain.

Notes and Suggestions

The methods to prevent spasm of calf muscles are:

(1) Gently and quickly knead and rub the muscles of the thigh with vibration using the proximal part of both palms. Work from the upper part of the thigh downward 6-12 times.

(2) Pinch and grasp the calf muscles with the fingers using activated qi from the top to the bottom of the leg; then press and knead the Yongquan (KI 1) point at the center of the sole of the foot using the thumb. Continue until a hot sensation is produced. This method can be used to prevent calf muscles spasms of athletes and workers who engage in heavy physical labour.

Case Report

Guo, a 15-year-old sportsman, first visited a clinic in April 1985 because of frequent painful spasms in the left calf muscles and limitation of movement in the leg after physical exhaustion or exposure to coldness at night. The patient also suffered from stretching pain in the ankle and toes when standing straight. After qigong therapy and application of external qi 6 times the calf muscle spasms were almost relieved; a hot and relaxing sensation was detected in the muscles.

Rheumatic Arthritis of the Knee Joint

Causes and Symptoms

This is an aching disease of the knee joint due to attacks of wind and dampness evils when patients are exposed to a cold and damp environment for a long time, dive into cold water right after profuse sweating or after an injury to their knee joint. Patients may suffer from aches in the knee joint and the surrounding ligaments; may impede walking and, in severe cases, reduce the knee jerk reflex. At chronic stages, patients may experience inflammation and swelling of the knee joints.

Techniques

Finger-pressing, pushing, rubbing and vibrating with activated qi and the routine qigong acupressure therapy for the lower limbs.

Treatment Procedure

(1) Finger-pressing: Patients take a supine posture. Apply the finger-pressing with activated qi to the Heding (EX-LE 2), Xiyan (EX-LE 5), Yanglingquan (GB 34) and Zusanli (ST 36) points and use the palm-pressing or vibration over the aching area to produce a penetrating, hot and relaxing sensation.

(2) Pushing and Rubbing: Patients take a supine posture. Push and rub the knee joint with the palm using activated qi to produce a penetrating, hot and relaxing

sensation.

(3) Vibrating: Patients lie on their stomach. Use the palm with activated qi to vibrate the back of the knee and use the finger to press the Weizhong (BL 40), Chengshan (BL 57) and Chengjin (BL 56) points to produce a hot sensation.

Notes and Suggestions

(1)Physical exercise of the hemoral quadriceps muscles may prevent contracture and rigidity of the knee joint.

(2) The knee joint should be well protected from external trauma and attacks of coldness and dampness.

(3) Patients should regularly perform the qigong exercises to strengthen their body resistance.

Case Report

Mr. He, a 62-year-old military officer, first visited a clinic in July 1986 with a 2-year history of rheumatic arthritis of the knee joints. The aching and swelling in the right knee was severe, and was aggravated by overcast and rainy weather. A physical examination showed a slight limitation of movement in the right knee joint, knocking pain and a positive floating test on the patella. A diagnosis of rheumatic arthritis of right knee joint was made. After qigong acupressure therapy with application of external qi 12 times, the pain and limitation of movement of his right knee joint was relieved. This treatment might produce a hot sensation in the knee joint.

Ankle Injuries

Causes and Symptoms

This is an acute sprain of the ankle joint with tearing of the articular ligaments, rupture of the capillary blood vessels, subcutaneous bleeding, swelling and bruising. This injury may interfere with ankle joint movement and, in severe cases, walking. If treatment is inadequate, the accumulated blood and soft tissue may be coagulated. The swelling and pain may last a long time and be combined with local chronic inflammation, impairment of blood circulation and functional disturbance.

Techniques

Finger-pressing, palm-pressing, stretching and vibrating combined with routine qigong acupressure therapy for the lower limbs.

Treatment Procedure

(1) Pushing and Pressing: Patients take a sitting posture. Put the thumb on the anterior side of outside the ankle and the index finger overlapped by the middle finger on the posterior side of inside the ankle to push and press the tendons with activated qi until a numb feeling is detected at the distal ends of toes.

(2) Pressing and Vibrating: Put the thumb on the anterior side of the ankle joint and the other four fingers behind the inside ankle joint to press with activated qi and vibrate the anterior joint space until a hot and numb sensation is detected in the big toe.

(3) Stretching and Vibrating: Use the fingers to pull the toes and at the same time to stretch and turn the instep of the injured foot outside. (This helps increase the medial articular space of the ankle joint.) Then use the thumb of the other hand to press the inner articular space. After that turn the instep of the injured foot inside and then use the thumb of the other hand to press the outside articular space. The vibrating with activated qi is applied to produce a localized hot and relaxing sensation.

Notes and Suggestions

(1) Vigorous kneading and grasping are contraindicated for acute ankle sprains with internal hemorrhage, but qigong acupressure therapy can be used to treat patients after internal bleeding has been controlled.

(2) The maneuvers should not be applied very vigorously; this would produce more damage in the injured joint.

(3) Qigong acupressure and the vibrating may cure chronic inflammation and injury of the ankle joint if the treatment can be sustained over a long enough period of time.

Case Report

Mr. Lin, a 50-year-old military officer, first visited a clinic in October 1986 because of an accidental sprain in the left ankle, which had happened three days before coming down the stairs. A physical examination showed swelling over the outside ankle joint, local tenderness and limitation of movement in the left ankle joint. After one qigong acupressure treatment with application of external qi, the pain in the joint was apparently reduced and the locomotive function was also improved. After 2 more treatments, the swelling and pain was entirely relieved and the normal movement of the ankle joint was almost restored.

Arm Sprains and Contusions

Causes and Symptoms

Sprains and contusions of the arm joints are an acute injury or a chronic strain of the shoulder, elbow, wrist and finger joints with pain, swelling and limitation of movement in the injured joints. The joints may become stiff and the muscles atrophic if the damaged joints can not be satisfactorily cured.

Diagnosis and Treatment

(1) Shoulder Sprains and Contusions: Qigong acupressure therapy for frozen shoulder may be used to treat this disease after you apply vibrating over the diseased area to promote blood circulation, resolve swelling and stop pain. This procedure will produce a hot sensation in the patient's shoulder.

(2) Elbow Sprains and Contusions: Apply the vibrating with activated qi over the elbow and then apply the pinching, grasping and gentle muscle-adjusting along the Hand-Yangming Meridian together with the finger-pressing (6-12 times) to remove blood stasis in the meridians and to stop pain.

(3) Wrist Sprains and Contusions: Apply the vibrating with activated qi to the

wrist and then direct the pressing and rubbing with pressure to the deep tissue underneath the acupoints, to produce a hot sensation. Pull, stretch, rotate and dorsiflex the injured wrist, with the five fingers of both the patient and the qigong practioner mutually crisscrossing each other to promote blood circulation, remove blood stasis from meridians and to stop pain.

(4) Finger Sprains and Contusions: Use vibrating with activated qi. Pull, rotate, shake and twist the injured fingers to correct the deformity. Vigorous acupressure treatment is detrimental to patients with torn tendons and ligaments. The injured finger may immobilized (bind it with a neighboring finger) for at least two weeks to facilitate healing of the tendons. Physical exercise should be carried on from the early stages of injury.

Techniques

Besides the therapeutic methods mentioned in above paragraph of diagnosis and treatment, finger-pressing, palm-pressing, kneading, twisting, pinching, stretching, bone-setting and vibrating with activated qi may also be adopted to treat the injury.

Case Report

Mr. Qian, a 35-year-old cadre from a company in Hebei Province, first visited a clinic in July 1984 because of a sprain of the left wrist by improperly lifting a heavy object 3 days before. The wrist was swollen and the pain was aggravated by rotation. After qigong acupressure therapy and application of external qi 2 times, the sprain was almost entirely relieved.

Lower Limb Sprains and Contusions

Causes and Symptoms

Sprain and contusion of the hip, knee, ankle and phalangeal joints of the lower limb are usually caused by acute trauma or chronic strain. Patients may suffer from bruises and swelling, pain and disturbance of articular movement.

Diagnosis and Treatment

(1) Hip Sprains and Contusions: This disease should be differentiated from hemoral neck fractures in aged people. Use the ulnar side of the hand to gently and slowly push and rub the injured area with activated qi; then pinch and grasp the lower limb from the hip region downward along the Foot-Yangming Meridian 6-12 times. It helps release meridian blockages, resolve swelling and stop pain.

(2) Knee Joint Sprains and Contusions: Use the palm with activated qi to rub the knee joint until a hot and relaxing sensation can be felt; then press the Xiyan (EX-LE 5) point. Vibrating with activated qi can be used to treat the accumulation of fluid in the knee joint. This help remove blood stasis from meridians, resolve swelling and stop pain.

(3) Ankle Sprains and Contusions: Use the palms with activated qi to gently push, press and rub the injured area in two directions; then flex the joint up and down and rub and twist the joint back and forth to reduce swelling, stop pain and release joint stiffness. For patients with torn ligaments, the joint should be immobilized with a

bandage to protect it and facilitate healing broken ligaments.

Techniques

Besides the methods mentioned in above paragraph, pushing, rubbing, twisting, kneading and stretching with activated qi can also be used to treat this disease.

Notes and Suggestions

(1) Injured ankle with ruptured ligaments should be immobilized to ensure ligament repair.

(2) In patients with subcutaneous hematoma the compression bandage should be applied first to the injured area and qigong acupressure therapy can be used until the hematoma has been absorbed.

Case Report

Mr. Gao, a 39-year-old manager from Guangzhou City, first visited a clinic in March 1986. Five days before visiting the clinic he acutely sprained his right big toe as he was getting off a train. The injured area was red, swollen and very painful; the sufferings were severely aggravated by walking. Although traditional massage is contraindicated for acute sprains with swelling, qigong acupressure therapy with external qi can be used to promote blood circulation, control inflammation and stop pain. After the qigong acupressure therapy with application of external qi 6 times, the injury of his big toe was completely cured.

Postencephalitis

Causes and Symptoms

Postencephalitis refers to complications that may arise from encephalitis; or brain inflammation. In traditional Chinese medicine this disease is caused by summer dampness evil. Cinical manifestations are very complicated and may be divided into three types:

(1) Patients may suffer from mental disturbance, apathy, depression, hyperactivity or restlessness and intellectural disturbance or amentia.

(2) Patients may suffer from dysphagia, aphasia, blindness, deafness, or slurred speech and impairment of vision and audition.

(3) Severe patients may suffer from spastic paralysis of the limbs; and opisthotonus, ataxia, paraplegia, general and local convulsion may appear in patients with transverse injury of the cervical spinal cord.

Techniques

Qigong acupuncture, Daoyin, patting and vibrating techniques.

Treatment Procedure

(1) Qigong Acupressure and Daoyin: Patients take a supine posture. Guide Dantian qi to the palm and induce it into the vertex of head [Baihui (DU 20)] to promote blood circulation, remove blood stasis and discharge turbid qi out of the body through the Yongquan (KI 1) point.

(2) Pinching and Nail-Pressing: Using your finger nail, slowly and rhythmically pinch and press the patient's base of fingernail and toenail pholangeal finger and toe

joints 6-12 times. In patients with deformities of the bilateral lower limbs, the hip joints are pulled apart from each other.

(3) Patting and Vibrating: Patting and vibrating with adequate force along the three meridian lines from the forehead to the occipital region of the head. This helps promote blood circulation and improve brain function; but the strong stimulation produced by this mothed may cause dizziness.

(4) Finger-Pressing at Acupoints: The acupoints are selected according to the symptoms of the patients:

Blindness: Neicishang [EX point, above Jingming (BL 1)], Jingming (BL 1) and Tongziliao (GB 1)

Deafness: Yifeng (SJ 17) and Tinggong (SI 19)

Abnormal Protrusion of the Tongue: Yifeng (SJ 17), Dicang (ST 4), Jiache (ST 6) and Hegu (LI 4)

Stiff Necks: Finger-pressing at Fengchi (GB 20) and physical exercise for the neck

Facial Paralysis: Same as the treatment for Bell's palsy.

Dysphagia: Finger-pressing at Tiantu (RN 22) and grasping and kneading applied at the sternocleidomastoid muscle.

For Functional Recovery of Joints: Besides qigong acupressure therapy, patients are encouraged to do active or passive physical exercise, such as leg-lifts, hip flexing, and leg extension, flexing, adduction and abduction exercises for the lower limbs; also, arm adduction, abduction, forward, backward and upward raising exercises; and elbow and wrist extension and flexing exercises for upper limb. At the same time, the Eight Pieces of Brocade Exercise (Chapter 3), breathing exercises for health maintenance and callisthenic exercises may be performed. Physical exercises for the upper limbs are more important in patients with hemiplegia; passive flexing exercising with the neck is prohibited in patients with stiff necks. For babies, exercise for paralyzed hands should be emphasized.

Speech and Intelligence Rehabilitation: This training should be started right after the recovery of consciousness. For example, teach and encourage the children to tell their name or to count numbers. For children with dysphonia teach them to speak by learning lip reading. In general, the qigong acupressure therapy may produce a satisfactory effect in patients with a short course of disease (less than 1 year), but the therapeutic result is poor in children with a long clinical course or those above 5 years old. Qigong acupressure therapy is contraindicated in patients with epilepsy.

Case Report

Ms. Hu, a 22-year-old telephone operator, first visited a clinic in December 1986 because of a 20-year history of encephalitis (suffered after a fever). The patient suffered from locomotive disturbance in the left limbs, spastic movement and an awkward gait, but her general condition was good. After 24 treatments of qigong acupressure therapy and application of external qi, the lower limb spasms were slightly relieved, the gait was smoother and the headache was alleviated.

Cerebral Palsy

Causes and Symptoms

Children with cerebral palsy may suffer from underdevelopment; leanness and weakness of the body and limbs; unsteady standing and walking; postponed tooth eruption; fine, sparse and yellow hair; apathy; and the inability to speak before 2-3 years old. This disease is due to bad health in pregnant mothers and congenital defects of the fetus or it can be caused by inadequate feeding or loss of diet regulation after birth. In cerebral palsy, the transporting and transforming function of the spleen is disturbed and the nutrition of food and drinks can not be distributed to enrich qi and blood.

Diagnosis and Treatment

(1) Delayed Growth of Hair: Induce qi to the central part of the palm until it becomes hot; then use the palm to press and rub the vertex of the child's head [Baihui (DU 20)], push the frontal and occipital hair line and apply vibration to release the blockage in the Yang Meridians and enhance the growth of hair. Repeat these 6-12 times.

(2) Postponed Tooth Eruption: Postponement in the eruption of deciduous teeth for 1 year or the postponement of permanent teeth for more than 1 year after the loss of deciduous teeth is due to insufficient kidney qi and spleen qi in the body. Therefore, pinching the muscles along the spine, kneading the loins and kidney regions, and rotational rubbing on the upper lip and lower jaw may be applied 6-12 times. This helps tonify and strengthen the kidney and to adjust the spleen and stomach.

(3) Retarded Speaking: Retardation of speech before 4-5 years old is due to a deficiency of heart qi and mental retardation. It can be differentiated from congenital deafness by the presence of hearing ability. Use the finger-pressing and kneading with activated qi along the cervical spinal column up to the posterior hair line, over the lower jaw and throat region and along the Taiyang and Yangming meridians from the shoulder through the arm to the tiger's mouth (part of the hand between the thumb and the forefinger) to strengthen the spleen, tonify the kidney, and increase intelligence. Repeat 6-12 times.

(4) Delayed Standing and Walking: For babies who can not stand and/or walk after 3-4 years old, use gentle pushing, pinching and grasping with activated qi on the lower limbs and the pulling on the phalangeal joints of the toes which will help tonify qi and blood, strengthen muscles and bones and tonify the liver and kidney. Do this 6-12 times. For children with weakness and tremor of the lower limbs, pressing and kneading may be applied over the sacral region [Baliao (BL 30-33) for 10-15 minutes.

(5) Underdevelopment of the Bones: Besides shortness of body stature and

weakness of physique, afflicted children also suffer from poor appetite, sallow complexion, lean musculature and flaccid limbs. Besides routine qigong acupressure therapy for the chest and abdomen, apply the nail-pressing and kneading with activated qi to the palmar side of the middle phalangeal joints of the fingers to adjust and tonify the stomach, strengthen the spleen and tonify the blood. Repeat 6-12 times.

Techniques

Besides the therapeutic methods mentioned in the above paragraph of diagnosis and treatment, pinching the muscles along the spine, finger-pressing, palm-pressing and rubbing with activated qi may also be adopted.

Notes and Suggestions

(1) The therapeutic effect of qigong acupressure therapy is satisfactory in the treatment of cerebral palsy. A therapeutic course contains 12 treatments; the second course may be started after a 7-15 day rest.

(2) The sick children should live a regular life and the food supply should be regular in time and in amount (neither too little or too much). Food should be rich in nutrition and not greasy.

(3) Finger-pressing with activated qi and kneading may be applied along the Du Meridian to promote circulation of meridianal qi, tonify the five organs and to increase disease resistance.

Case Report

Zheng, a boy of three and a half years old, suffered from cerebral palsy caused by hypoxia during birth. Clinical manifestations showed the functional disturbance of the bilateral lower limbs (more severe on the right side), inability to sit and stand, blurred speech and drooling. After 24 treatments of qigong acupressure therapy and application of external qi, the drooling was improved and his speech became more clearer; after 48 treatments the boy could sit up and walk slowly with a slight support. His general health was also much improved.

Hemiplegia

Causes and Symptoms

Among many causal factors, cerebral accidents (strokes), including cerebral hemorrhages due to hypertension and arterosclerosis, cerebral thrombosis, cerebral embolism and cerebral arterial spasm, is the most common cause of hemiplegia. Head injuries and intracranial tumors may also produce this disease. According to traditional Chinese medicine theory, it is caused by an excess of liver yang and imbalance between yin and yang due to worrying, anger, overeating, alcoholism, emotional disturbance, excessive phlegm and dampness and deficiency of vital energy. Patients may suffer from a sudden fall and loss of consciousness, hemiplegia, facial paralysis, drooling, slurred speech or aphasia. In acute stages the paralysis is flaccid in nature; in late stages it is spastic. Patients may show muscular spasms, clenched fists and tightly flexed elbow joints. Spastic lower limbs may be stretched straight, knee joints stiff. Also, the ankle joints collapsed and their dorsiflexion function is impaired, causing a laterally circling gait.

Techniques

Qigong acupressure therapy, Daoyin and massage techniques with activated qi are used to treat hemiplegic patients.

Treatment Procedure

(1) Qigong Acupressure Therapy and Daoyin: Patients take a supine or sitting posture. Activate and move Dantian qi to the inner Laogong (PC 8) point on the palm and then put the palm over the vertex of the head [Baihui (DU 20)] to Daoyin qi into the patient's body. This helps discharge turbid qi out of the body through the Yongquan (KI 1) point for adjusting qi and blood and releasing meridian blockages.

(2) Finger-Pressing at Acupoints: Patients take a supine posture. Move Dantian qi to both hands and use the finger to press the acupoints on the meridian from the distal end to the proximal end of the affected limb.

(3) Functional Exercise of Joints: Patients should perform active and passive physical exercise to improve movement in the four limbs. With assistance from another person, the patient may sit up in bed, stand up, and walk. Physical exercise can promote blood circulation, improve joint movement, prevent the development of deformity and restore normal locomotive function.

(4) Supplemental Treatment: For aphasia with impaired movement of the tongue, use the index and middle fingers with activated qi to press the root of tongue for 3-5 minutes and to pull the tongue out of the mouth. At the same time, use the finger-pressing technique at Yingxiang (LI 20), Sibai (ST 2), Chengjiang (RN 24) and Yamen (DU 15).

For aphonia due to paralysis of the facial muscles, finger-pressing may be applied at Tiantu (RN 22), Renying (ST 9), Jiache (ST 6) and Hegu (LI 4).

For facial paralysis: Refer to the treatment of Bell's facial palsy.

Notes and Suggestions

(1) Emergent Treatment: Patients should not be moved or transported right after acute attacks, if not indicated and they should be confined to their beds for absolute rest and their respiration, pulse, pupils, consciousness and body temperature should be carefully monitored. Blood pressure should be appropriately adjusted in stroke patients with hypertension. In patients with mild cerebral hemorrhaging or with subcortical bleeding, 6-aminoacetic acid and dicynone may be administered. If the hemorrhage can not be controlled or it happens in the cerebellum, surgical operation may be done to save the patient's life.

(2) Prevention of Complications: At acute stages, infection of the upper respiratory tract and urinary system and the development of bedsores should be carefully prevented. At the same time, normal function of joints should be well maintained. To prevent contraction and deformity in these limbs, their positions should be changed several times in a day.

Case Reports

(1) Mr. Zheng, a 53-year-old patient from Taiwan, first visited a clinic in

September 1986 with a 2-year history of hemiplegia after cerebral embolism. A physical examination showed leanness, impaired locomotive function in the left limbs, limited flexibility in the left ankle and slurred speech. A diagnosis of hemiplegia after cerebral accident was made. After 24 treatments of qigong acupressure therapy with application of external qi, his speech and walking were improved and his muscular strength increased. After further treatments, other symptoms were also much improved.

(2) Mr. Wang, a 42-year-old associate professor, had strokes in 1985 and 1986 with a sequela of hemiplegia. The patient suffered from locomotive dysfunction of the right limbs, severe hand tremors, lameness, ataxia, constant dizziness and headaches. His blood pressure was 190/100 mm Hg. After 24 treatments of qigong acupressure therapy with application of external qi, his muscular strength in the lower limbs was increased and he could walk more and more steadily. After the treatments, his hand tremors (which had troubled him for 9 months and hindered his ability to grasp objects and to write) were nearly under control and he could write again. His general symptoms were also improved.

(3) Mrs. Liang, age 52, had hemiplegia for 5 years. The patient could not take care of her own daily life. She was taken to a clinic on a stretcher. After 12 treatments of qigong acupressure therapy with application of external qi, the patient could raise her paralyzed leg and after 24 treatments, she could walk a few steps. At the same time, her general symptoms were also improved.

Traumatic Paraplegia

Causes and Symptoms
Paraplegia is usually caused by damage to the spinal cord due to fracture or dislocation of the spinal column after trauma. Patients may show a series of clinical manifestations, including motor and sensory disturbance and incontinence of urine and stools. The symptoms vary with the location, severity and range of the injury. If treatment and nursing care are not adequate and effective, patients may develop complications, such as bedsores, infection of the urinary tract and enteroparalysis. According to traditional Chinese medicine theory, paraplegia is caused by the poor nutrition of the skin, muscles, tendons and bones due to exhaustion of *jinye* (body fluid) of the internal organs (caused by heat evil or due to deficiency of *jinye* of stomach after blockage of the Yangming Meridian by heat evil; and it may also be caused by the damage of the Du Meridian and dysfunction of the Dai (girdle) Meridian resulting from external traumas such as falling down.

Techniques
Finger-pressing, palm-pressing and kneading with activated qi together with physical exercise for functional recovery.

Treatment Procedure
(1) Finger-pressing and Daoyin: Patients take a supine posture and relax their body. Move Dantian qi to the palm and put it over the vertex of the patient's head

[Baihui (DU 20)] to lead qi into the patient's body to drive turbid qi out of the body through Yongquan (KI 1). At the same time, lead qi to the limbs to promote blood circulation and improve locomotive function in the joints.

(2) Pressing and Kneading: Patients lie on their back and relax. Move Dantian qi to the palm and use it to press and knead the limbs along the meridians (from the distal end to the proximal end of the limbs).

(3) Finger-Pressing: Patients lie on their stomach or on their healthy side. Move qi to both palms and put one palm over Dazhui (DU 14) and another palm over Mingmen (DU 4) to regulate bodily functions. Then use finger-pressing, kneading and patting along the spinal column and Urinary Bladder Meridian from the upper to the lower part of the body.

(4) Exercises for Joints: Patients take a supine posture. Guide them through active and passive physical exercise. At the beginning, do exercises to raise the hips from the bed and stretch the back, as well as sit-ups. Later on, patients may stand up and bear some weight, walking with a slight support from another person. Physical exercise may promote blood circulation, prevent deformity and enhance functional recovery of joints.

Diagnosis and Treatment

(1) Stool and Urine Incontinence: Apply the finger-pressing with activated qi at the ischial tuberosity, Gunei (EX point, medial surface of the thigh), Chipang (EX point, beside the pubic symphysis), Qugu (RN 2), Shenshu (BL 23), Zusanli (ST 36), Sanyinjiao (SP 6) and Yanglingquan (GB 34). With concentrated awareness, do abdominal breathing with the arms dropped down during expiration and with the palms slowly pressed over the lower abdomen. This will produce a numb, swelling and hot sensation in the urethra.

(2) Reduced Abdominal Muscle Tension: Patting with activated qi is applied over the abdominal wall.

(3) Stool Incontinence: Pressing and strumming with activated qi are applied at Yaoyan (EX-B 7), Pishu (BL 20), Dachangshu (BL 25), Shenque (RN 8), Guanyuan (RN 4) and Tianshu (ST 25).

(4) Urine Incontinence with Reduced Abdominal Muscle Tension: Patting with activated qi is applied over the abdominal wall. The mind is concentrated at the Dantian and the patient does abdominal breathing. Patting is applied over the abdominal wall during inhalation and stopped during expiration. At the beginning, the abdomen is gently patted 8-12 times; the force and times of patting may be gradually increased.

(5) Exercise and Self-Treatment with Qigong Acupressure Therapy: The following exercises and treatment may be selected according to the severity of paralysis, functional disturbance and general condition of the patient:

Spastic Paraplegia: Patients perform relaxation exercises and static inner-health cultivation exercises. Gentle qigong acupressure therapy and massage may be used to do self-treatment.

Flaccid Paraplegia: Patients employ physical and breathing exercises with conduction of qi. Moderate qigong acupressure therapy and massage may be used to do self-treatment.

For Patients with a Grade 0 Myodynamia of Paralytic Lower Limbs: Passive therapeutic exercises may be applied to each joint of the paralytic limbs and the patients should use their minds to create imaginary muscular contraction.

For Patients with a Grade 1-2 Myodynamia of Paralytic Lower Limbs: Physical and breathing exercises with concentration of mind should be done. Patients are taught to transfer qi to the paralytic limbs to promote the circulation of the blood. Because of weak muscles, patients may need help and support to carry on physical exercise.

For Patients with a Grade 3 Myodynamia of Paralytic Lower Limbs: Patients are encouraged to do active physical exercise for each joint of the limbs and to perform self-massage for health. If the patients can stand up, they are advised to do the Shaolin Post-Standing exercise (Chapter 2) and gradually increasing the duration.

For Patients with a Grade 4 Myodynamia of Paralytic Lower Limbs: Patients should do physical exercise to improve muscle strength by doing Sinew-Transforming exercise, Taijiquan, Eight Pieces of Brocade Exercise or Calisthenic Exercise (Chapter 3).

For Patients with Infection and Functional Disturbance in the Urinary System: The patients may perform microcosmic oribit circulating exercises with attention concentrated at the lower Dantian. In addition, they are encouraged to drink plenty of water to control the infection.

Case Report

Mrs. Yao, a 38-year-old worker from Shaanxi Province, first visited a clinic in November 1986 with a history of compressive bone fracture of 11th and 12th thoracic vertebrae. The patient could not sit up in bed and she suffered from numbness, pain and muscular atrophy of both lower limbs; also, general weakness and incontinence of urine and stools. A diagnosis of paraplegia after compressive bone fracture of the 11th and 12th thoracic vertebrae was made. After 4 treatments of qigong acupressure therapy with application of external qi, the patient could turn over on bed; after 12 treatments, she could perform physical exercise in a wheel chair; and after 24 treatments, the patient regained urination sensations. EMG determinations and skin sensation tests also showed some improvement.

Bed-Wetting (Enuresis)

Causes and Symptoms

This disease is caused by latent epilepsy, dysfunction of the urinary bladder sphinctors, mental hyperirritability due to phimosis, balantitis and infection of pinworm. In some children, it is caused by congenital spina bifida. Bed-wetting usually happens at night after falling asleep (with or without dreams of urination). The children may suddenly wake up or continue to sleep until the next morning.

Urination during the daytime is normal.

Techniques

Qigong acupressure therapy and pinching the muscles along the spine.

Treatment Procedure

(1) Finger-pressing at Acupoints: Patients lie on their backs. Do finger-pressing with activated qi at Sanyinjiao (SP 6), Pishu (BL 20), Weishu (BL 21), Sanjiaoshu (BL 22) and Mingmen (DU 4) points 3-6 times until a tense and hot sensation can be felt in the lower abdomen.

(2) Pinching Along the Spine: Pinching along the spinal column from the level of Changqiang (DU 1) upward to the level of Dazhui (DU 14) 6-12 times to remove stagnation in the meridians, adjust function of internal organs, tonify qi and blood and enhance body resistance.

Case Report

Li, a 6-year-old boy, was first brought to a clinic in March 1983 with a 2-year history of enuresis. He often wet his bed after falling asleep soundly at night, and it would not be discovered until the next morning. After qigong acupressure therapy with application of external qi was used to treat him once a day for 6 days, the frequence of bed-wetting was reduced; after 6 more treatments, the bed-wetting was almost cured.

Infantile Indigestion

Causes and Symptoms

Infantile indigestion, also called infantile diarrhea, usually occurs in the summer and autumn. It is a common disease in babies below 2 years old. The mild type is called infantile indigestion and the severe type is known as toxic indigestion. This disease is usually caused by damage and dysfunction of the spleen and stomach due to inadequate feeding, intake of unhealthy food or due to attacks of summer dampness. Afflicted babies may have frequent diarrhea, passing thin, pastelike or yolklike stools with mucus. In addition, they may have nausea and vomiting, and their body temperature may be normal or slightly elevated. Babies with the severe type may suffer from repeated vomiting, lassitude, restlessness, pale complexion, cherry-colored lips, deep respiration, sunken eye socket, reduced skin elasticity, oligouria or anuria. Babies with severe dehydration may develop shock and convulsion.

Techniques

Routine qigong acupressure therapy and finger-pressing, palm-pressing, pushing, rubbing techniques and pinching the muscles along the spine.

Treatment Procedure

(1) Babies are held in their parent's arm or put in a semi-recumbent position. Move qi to the palm until a hot feeling is detected there; with the palm, push and grasp the chest and abdomen of the baby and do rotational rubbing around the umbilicus. Then, routine acupressure therapy is applied 6-12 times to promote blood circulation and enhance intestinal peristalsis.

(2) Apply the finger-pressing at the acupoints beside the spinal column over the back and lower back. Kneading from the upper part of the back downward. For babies with frequent diarrhea a finger with activated qi is used to press Guiwei (EX point) and another finger with activated qi is used to push (upward) Changqiang (DU 1) and to deliver qi to restore the potency of the Du Meridian, promote circulation of qi and blood and to adjust internal organ function.

(3) Apply finger-pressing with activated qi to bilateral Zusanli (ST 36) and bilateral Neiguan (PC 6) 6-12 times. This helps strengthen the spleen, tonify qi, warm up yang and stop diarrhea.

Notes and Suggestions

(1) Qigong acupressure therapy is very useful in the treatment of infantile diarrhea and especially effective in babies with frequent diarrhea. The symptoms can be gradually alleviated and relieved.

(2) Pinching the muscles along the spine should be applied in the early morning and before the breakfast, but not after a big meal. After this treatment the babies should be put in a bed to have a rest before having breakfast. In addition, measures to maintain food hygiene, preserve body warmth and prevent common cold should be earnestly adopted for babies.

(3) Throughout the therapeutic course, babies should be carefully watched for early diagnosis and urgent treatment of toxic infantile diarrhea. Because of the serious loss of body fluids, babies may have sunken eye socket, dryness of oral mucosa and skin, restlessness or drowsiness.

Case Report

Li, a 2-year-old boy, was first brought to a clinic in September 1978 because of a half-year-long history of difficult feeding, nausea, vomiting and diarrhea. The baby passed loose and flaky stools with mucus 7-8 times a day; he also showed sallow complexion, leanness, lassitude, abdominal distension, constant crying and restlessness. After 6 treatments of qigong acupressure therapy with application of external qi, the symptoms of indigestion were quickly alleviated; after 10 treatments, the above-mentioned symptoms were almost entirely relieved.

Myogenic Torticollis in Children

Causes and Symptoms

It is usually due to injury of the neck muscles caused by compression of the birth canal or obstetric forceps in the birth process. This disease can be divided into the forced contracture type and the flaccid type. The contracture of muscles is due to the hematoma (blood blockages and swelling) caused by injury; or due to the paralysis of the neck muscles after childhood febrile diseases. A long lump can be found on one side of the neck on a newborn baby and it may spontaneously disappear a half-year later. The head of the baby may favor turning to the normal side while the neck leaning to the injured side. In flaccid torticollis the head of the baby may favor turning to one side. In late stages, the child may develop scoliosis of the thoracic spinal column.

Techniques

Pushing, kneading, pinching, grasping, palm-vibrating, stretching and pulling with activated qi.

Treatment Procedure

(1) Patients are put in a sitting position. Push and knead the involved muscles 6-12 times, then to pinch and grasp the nape of the neck and scapular muscles, and the arm along the hand Shaoyang Meridian and finally to do finger-pressing at Hegu (LI 4).

(2) Holds the patient's shoulder on the diseased side with one hand. Push the head with another hand toward the normal side to stretch the damaged muscles 6-12 times; then gently flex the neck forward and backward with the neck under traction; and finally use the side of the hand with activated qi to push the neck and nape region with vibration.

(3) The treatment is given once a day or every 2 days and a therapeutic course contains 12 treatments. The second course may be started after a 1-week rest.

Notes and Suggestions

Qigong acupressure therapy, along with neck exercises, may produce a satisfactory result.

Case Report

Wang, a 4-year-old boy, was brought to a clinic in July 1985 to treat his torticollis of the left side of the neck. Past treatments given in other hospitals all failed because of the poor cooperation of the child. A physical examination showed a lump palpable on the left side of the neck and head movement was limited. After 12 treatments of qigong acupressure therapy with application of external qi, the neck deformity was apparently corrected and the symptoms were almost completely relieved.

图书在版编目(CIP)数据

中华气功点穴疗法精粹:英文/黄孝宽编著.

—北京:外文出版社,1997

ISBN 7 - 119 - 00748 - 3

Ⅰ.中… Ⅱ.黄… Ⅲ.穴位按压疗法:气功疗法－中国－英文 Ⅳ.R244.1

中国版本图书馆 CIP 数据核字 (96) 第 12874 号

责任编辑　张纬雯

封面设计　朱振安

中华气功点穴疗法精粹

黄孝宽编著

*

ⓒ外文出版社

外文出版社出版

(中国北京百万庄大街 24 号)

邮政编码 100037

北京外文印刷厂印刷

中国国际图书贸易总公司发行

(中国北京车公庄西路 35 号)

北京邮政信箱第 399 号　邮政编码 100044

1997 年(16 开)第 1 版

1997 年第 1 版第 1 次印刷

(英)

ISBN 7 - 119 - 00748 - 3 /R·21(外)

05500

14 - E - 3097S